Chest, Heart and Vascular Disorders for Physiotherapists

Chest, Heart and Vascular Disorders for Physiotherapists

Edited by
JOAN E. CASH
B.A., F.C.S.P., Dip.T.P.

FABER AND FABER
3 Queen Square
London

First published in 1975
by Faber and Faber Limited
3 Queen Square London WC1

Reprinted 1975 and 1977

Printed in Great Britain by
Whitstable Litho Ltd, Whitstable, Kent
All rights reserved

ISBN 0 571 10618 8 (paper covers)
ISBN 0 571 10412 6 (hard bound edition)

Acknowledgements

Miss Beazley would like to thank the physiotherapy teaching staff, particularly Mr. J. O. Jenkins, M.C.S.P., Dip.T.P., Mrs. D. Till, M.C.S.P., Dip.T.P. and Miss M. Farmer, M.C.S.P., Dip.T.P. and students of St. Mary's Hospital, Paddington, who have read her chapters and given helpful suggestions; her thanks also go to the American Heart Association through the office of their Assistant Medical Director, Ezra Lamden, M.D., for their help.

Miss Gaskell wishes to thank Dr. D. A. Ryland, M.R.C.P., for all his help and guidance with writing her chapters. Figures 5/2 to 5/6 are adapted by permission of the Brompton Hospital, London, and Figure 5/1 by permission of the Cystic Fibrosis Research Trust.

Miss Innocenti wishes to thank those who have helped in the preparation of her chapters, especially Mr. R. J. Cooper, Principal of the School of Physiotherapy, Guy's Hospital, and members of the Surgical Thoracic Unit and the photographic department of Guy's Hospital.

Miss Pickering would like to express her sincere thanks to Mr. H. H. G. Eastcott, M.S., who taught her so much when she was working for him, and for giving her so much help. She would also like to thank the staff of the Medical School Library and Miss Wigham and the staff of the physiotherapy department of St. Mary's Hospital, Paddington, for their help and tolerance while she was preparing her chapters.

Miss Waddington would like to thank Dr. Trevor B. Stretton, F.R.C.P., Consultant Physician, Miss B. Newton, S.R.N., Sister-in-Charge, Respiratory Care Unit, Miss E. H. Eaton, M.C.S.P., Dip.T.P., Miss J. Nicholas, M.C.S.P. and Miss S. Brown, M.C.S.P., all from Manchester Royal Infirmary, for their help in the preparation of her chapters. Figure 1/4 is reproduced by kind permission

Acknowledgements

of the authors, Dr. A. F. Foster-Carter and Dr. G. Simon, and the editor of *Thorax*.

Miss Cash feels very greatly indebted to the authors of the different sections of this book for their hard work and valuable contributions.

Miss Cash would also like to take this opportunity of expressing very sincere thanks to Mrs. Audrey Besterman, medical artist, and Miss P. Jean Cunningham, Editor of Nursing and Medical Books, and Miss Heather Potter, Assistant Editor, Faber & Faber Ltd., for the tremendous amount of work and for the interest and the care they have shown in the final preparation of the book.

Contents

Contents

Figures

11

Figures

Figures

Contributors

Miss E. A. Beazley, M.C.S.P., DIP.T.P.,
Assistant Principal,
School of Physiotherapy,
St. Mary's Hospital,
London, W.2.

Cardiac Conditions

Miss D. V. Gaskell, M.C.S.P.,
Superintendent Physiotherapist,
Brompton Hospital,
London, S.W.3.

Pulmonary Disease

Miss D. M. Innocenti, M.C.S.P.,
Superintendent Physiotherapist,
Physiotherapy Department,
Guy's Hospital,
London, S.E.1.

Thoracic Surgery

Miss J. Pickering, M.C.S.P.,
Senior Physiotherapist,
Physiotherapy Department,
St. Mary's Hospital,
London, W.2.

Peripheral Vascular Disease

Miss P. J. Waddington, M.C.S.P., H.T., DIP.T.P.,
Teacher,
The School of Physiotherapy,
The United Manchester Hospitals,
Manchester Royal Infirmary.

Anatomy and
Physiology of Respiration
and Intensive Care

CHAPTER 1

Outline of Anatomy of the Respiratory System

by P. J. WADDINGTON, M.C.S.P., H.T., DIP.T.P.

THE THORACIC CAVITY

The thoracic cage is formed by a bony framework consisting of the twelve thoracic vertebrae, twelve pairs of ribs and their costal cartilages and the sternum.

The thorax is kidney-shaped in cross-section because the ribs extend backwards beyond the plane of the vertebral column before arching forwards. The most posterior part of each rib, the angle, can be identified by an oblique ridge on the external surface. From the angle the rib is directed obliquely downwards and forwards. The degree of this obliquity increases progressively from the first to the ninth rib inclusive, after which the tendency is reversed. The seventh rib is the longest.

Posteriorly the head of a typical rib articulates with demi-facets on the bodies of its numerically equal thoracic vertebra and the one above, as well as with the intervening intervertebral disc, to form a synovial plane joint. The first, tenth, eleventh and twelfth ribs are atypical in articulating with the body of only one vertebra. The tubercles of the upper ten ribs also articulate with the transverse processes of their numerically equal vertebrae forming synovial plane joints.

Anteriorly, of the twelve pairs of ribs the first seven articulate with the sternum and are called vertebrosternal or true ribs. The costal cartilage of the first rib is joined directly to the sternum, forming a synchondrosis, whereas the costal cartilages of the other true ribs form synovial joints with the sternum. The eighth, ninth and tenth

17

ribs articulate with the costal cartilage of the rib above and are called vertebrochondral ribs; the last two pairs are free and are tipped with costal cartilage. They are called vertebral or floating ribs. The lower five pairs together as a group are called false ribs.

The sternum has three parts, from above downwards, the manubrium sterni, the corpus sterni or body and the small xiphoid process. The first costal cartilage articulates with the manubrium. The second articulates at the sternal angle or manubriosternal junction which is easily palpable through the skin as a ridge and is the most reliable point from which to identify the ribs and their costal cartilages. The remaining true ribs articulate with the body of the sternum, the last two (sixth and seventh) with its inferior border.

The gaps between adjacent ribs, or the intercostal spaces, are filled by the intercostal muscles. These are arranged in three layers like the flat muscles of the abdominal wall and their fibres follow a similar direction. Contraction of these muscles effects rib movement and prevents indrawing and bulging of the intercostal spaces due to changes of intrathoracic pressure during inspiration and expiration. The thoracic vessels and nerves are segmental in distribution and follow the line of each rib, lying between the middle and innermost layers of the intercostal muscles and membranes.

The thoracic inlet or upper opening of the thorax is formed by the body of the first thoracic vertebra, the first pair of ribs and their costal cartilages and the upper part of the manubrium sterni. It measures approximately 5 cm in an anteroposterior direction and 10 cm transversely.

The thoracic outlet or lower boundary of the thorax is formed by the body of the twelfth thoracic vertebra, the last pair of ribs, the lower six costal cartilages and the xiphoid process.

The thoracic cavity is divided from the abdominal cavity by a dome-shaped sheet of muscle and fibrous tissue, the diaphragm. The muscle fibres of this take origin from the perimeter of the thoracic outlet and converge to be inserted into a thin trefoil-shaped aponeurosis, the central tendon, which lies just below the pericardium and blends with it. When relaxed the diaphragm at its highest point rises to the level of the fifth and sixth ribs, being slightly higher on the right than on the left. It will be seen that as well as protecting the contents of the thorax itself, the thoracic cage protects the upper abdominal viscera, *i.e.* the liver, the stomach and the spleen.

The thoracic cavity is divided into three parts, the right and left pleural cavities and the region in between which is called the mediastinum.

The Pleura

Each pleura consists of two layers which are continuous with each other. The lung is surrounded by it rather as if a clenched fist were pressed into a partially inflated balloon. The wrist represents the root of the lung which is formed by structures entering or leaving the lung at the hilum (the area on the mediastinal surface of the lung through which structures enter and leave the lung), that is the bronchus, the pulmonary artery and the two pulmonary veins, the bronchial arteries and veins and the pulmonary plexus of nerves and lymph vessels.

The outer layer or parietal pleura lines the thoracic cavity and is attached to it. The inner visceral layer or pulmonary pleura covers the entire surface of the lungs entering into the fissures and covering the inter-lobar surfaces. The two layers lie one against the other and are lubricated by a thin layer of pleural fluid.

During inspiration the thoracic cage lined by the parietal pleura is enlarged, the lungs covered by the pulmonary pleura expand and air enters. Therefore as inspiration is followed by expiration and so on, there is a continuous sliding of the pulmonary pleura on the parietal pleura.

The parietal pleura is named according to the structures which it covers, thus, the costal pleura covers the ribs, the diaphragmatic pleura the diaphragm, and the mediastinal pleura the mediastinum, starting at the root of the lung. The part of the pleura from the root of the lung extending almost to the diaphragm is called the pulmonary ligament. The cervical pleura extends into the neck through the thoracic inlet.

The Lungs

The lungs occupying the pleural cavities are not identical in size and shape. The left lung is slightly smaller because the heart and pericardium lie more to the left of mid-line than to the right: this modification in the shape of the left lung which accommodates the heart is called the cardiac notch. The right lung, although it is the larger, is slightly shorter because the dome of the diaphragm is slightly raised on that side.

Each lung is divided into two by an oblique fissure which extends

19

into the lung almost as far as the hilum. A line drawn from the third thoracic vertebra posteriorly to the sixth costochondral junction, at which level it reaches the lower border of the lungs, represents the surface marking of the oblique fissure. The part of the lung below this fissure is called the lower lobe. Above the oblique fissure the right lung is divided again by a horizontal fissure extending forwards from the oblique fissure in the axillary line to the fourth costal cartilage (see Fig. 1/1). Thus an upper lobe is formed above the horizontal fissure and a middle lobe is formed below. The left lung is not subdivided in this way and the whole section is called the upper lobe. The antero-inferior part of the left upper lobe (equivalent to the middle lobe on the right) is called the lingula.

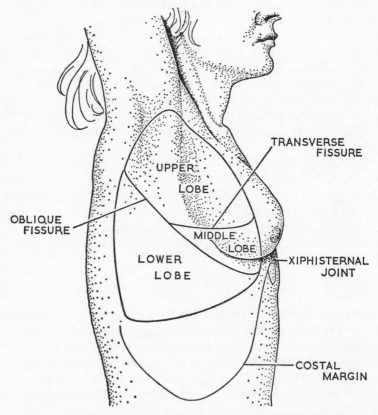

FIG. 1/1. Surface projection of the fissures and lobes of the right lung

Thus each lower lobe forms the base and the posterior portion of the entire lung and each upper or upper and middle lobes comprise the apex and anterior portion.

The lungs are of a spongy consistency and would be pink in colour were it not for atmospheric pollution.

Mediastinum

The space in the centre of the thoracic cavity between the pleural sacs is called the mediastinum. On either side it is covered by the mediastinal pleura and it extends from the thoracic inlet above to the diaphragm below and from the sternum anteriorly to the bodies of the thoracic vertebrae posteriorly. It contains the heart, the great vessels entering and leaving the heart, the oesophagus, the trachea and its bifurcation, the phrenic and vagus nerves, the thoracic duct and many lymph nodes.

For ease of description the mediastinum is divided into two parts by a horizontal plane joining the sternal angle (second costal carti-lage) to the lower border of the body of the fourth thoracic vertebra. The superior mediastinum lies above and the inferior mediastinum below this imaginary plane which passes through the bifurcation of the trachea and the concavity of the aortic arch.

The heart lies in the inferior mediastinum. Behind it and separating it from the bodies of the fifth to the eighth thoracic vertebrae lie the oesophagus and the descending aorta. The oesophagus leaves the thorax by piercing the diaphragm at the level of the body of the tenth thoracic vertebra and the aorta leaves the thorax without piercing the diaphragm by passing behind the median arcuate ligament at the level of the twelfth thoracic vertebra.

Deoxygenated blood enters the right atrium via the superior vena cava, which drains the upper half of the body, the inferior vena cava which carries blood from below the diaphragm and the coronary sinus which drains the myocardium. The superior vena cava begins at the level of the first right costal cartilage adjacent to the sternum and ends opposite the third right costal cartilage. It is formed by the junction of the two brachiocephalic veins and enters the upper part of the atrium. The inferior vena cava, which is formed by the junction of the common iliac veins, ascends on the right of the vertebral bodies and enters the mediastinum by passing through the diaphragm level with the lower border of the eighth thoracic vertebra and continues upwards, piercing the pericardium, to enter the lower part of the right atrium.

After passing through the tricuspid valve into the right ventricle the deoxygenated blood leaves the heart, passing through the pulmonary valve into the pulmonary trunk. At the level of the fifth thoracic vertebra the pulmonary trunk divides into the right and left pulmonary arteries each of which enters the corresponding lung at the hilum.

Oxygenated blood leaves the lungs and is carried in four pulmonary veins, two from each lung. After piercing the pericardium they open into the left atrium. Having passed into the left ventricle through the mitral valve, the blood leaves the heart via the aorta which originates at the aortic valve. The aorta ascends towards the manubrium and passes over the left bronchus before arching backwards towards the body of the fourth thoracic vertebra. The arch of the aorta lies within the superior mediastinum and connects the ascending aorta with the descending aorta which begins at the lower border of the fourth thoracic vertebra. Branches from the aorta supply the heart (coronary arteries), the lungs (bronchial arteries) and the whole of the systemic circulation.

THE RESPIRATORY PASSAGES

The respiratory passages, which carry air from the atmosphere to the alveoli, consist of the nose and mouth, the pharynx, the larynx, the trachea and the two main bronchi and their branches within the lungs. It is essential that these should remain open; they are therefore supported by either bone or cartilage as far as the bronchioles (see Fig. 1/2).

The Nose

The nose is divided into two cavities by the nasal septum, formed of thin bone (vomer and ethmoid) and cartilage. The base is provided by the hard palate and the roof mainly by the cribriform plate of the ethmoid bone. The lateral walls are undulating, being crossed in a horizontal direction by three pieces of bone, like the crests of waves, the superior, middle and inferior conchae, which are separated from each other by troughs, the superior, middle and inferior meatuses. The paranasal sinuses, the frontal, maxillary, ethmoidal and

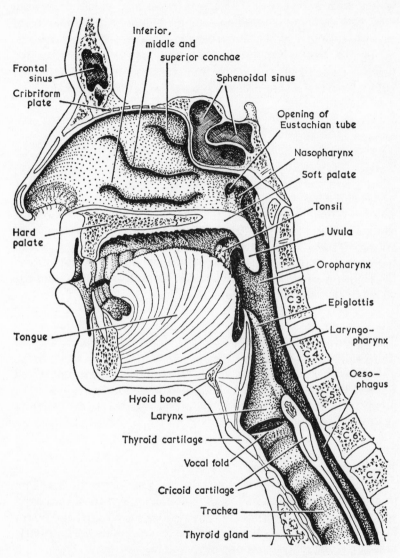

FIG. 1/2. A sagittal section through the nasal and oral cavities, pharynx and larynx

sphenoidal, lie within the bones of the skull and open into the lateral wall of each nasal cavity. The nasal cavities and the air sinuses are lined with columnar ciliated epithelium. Anteriorly, where the nasal cavities are open to the atmosphere, lie the nostrils protected by bristle-like hairs. Posteriorly each nasal cavity opens into the pharynx. The opening is called the posterior naris and measures approximately 2·5 cm (vertically) by 1·25 cm (horizontally).

The Pharynx

The pharynx is a fibromuscular funnel-shaped cavity about 15 cm long. It is divided into three parts.

THE NASOPHARYNX

This lies behind the nasal cavities. The roof is formed by bones of the skull. It lies above the soft palate which divides it from the other parts of the pharynx during swallowing. The auditory or eustachian tubes open one into each side of the nasopharynx, connecting it with the tympanic cavities. This regulates the air pressure on the two sides of the tympanic membranes.

THE OROPHARYNX

This lies behind the mouth, below the soft palate and extends as far down as the larynx.

The tonsils are two masses of lymphoid tissue lying in the lateral walls of the oropharynx. They form part of a circular band of lymphoid tissue which acts as a filter, protecting the respiratory tract against infection.

THE LARYNGOPHARYNX

This lies behind the larynx.

Air enters the nose, passes into the nasopharynx and from there through the oropharynx and finally into the upper part of the larynx and trachea. These upper respiratory pathways have three important functions: filtering and humidifying the inspired air and, if necessary, raising its temperature to body temperature.

This region has a very rich blood supply.

24

The Larynx

The larynx extends from the level of the third cervical vertebra to the lower border of the sixth cervical vertebra and lies between the pharynx above and the trachea below. The shape of the larynx is maintained by two hyaline and elastic cartilages, the thyroid and the cricoid. The thyroid cartilage or Adam's apple consists of two laminae which are fused together anteriorly in mid-line. The cricoid cartilage forms the only complete ring of cartilage, being wider posteriorly than anteriorly. It lies below the thyroid cartilage which fits over it to form two synovial joints. The arytenoid cartilages are two small pyramidal structures which lie interiorly and articulate with the upper posterior border of the cricoid cartilage. The paired

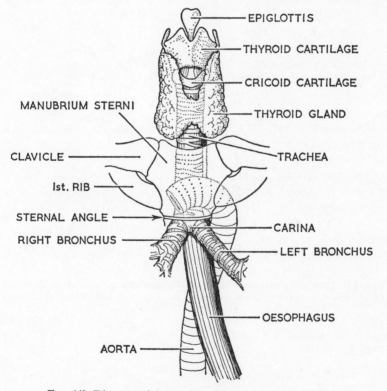

FIG. 1/3. Diagram of the trachea showing its main relations

Outline of Anatomy of the Respiratory System

Right Lung	
Upper Lobe {	1. Apical
	2. Posterior
	3. Anterior
Middle Lobe {	4. Lateral
	5. Medial

Left Lung	
Upper Lobe {	1. ⎫
	2. ⎬ Apico-posterior
	3. Anterior
	4. Superior ⎫ Lingular
	5. Inferior ⎭

Right Lung	
Lower Lobe {	6. Apical
	7. Medial basal
	8. Anterior basal
	9. Lateral basal
	10. Posterior basal

Left Lung	
Lower Lobe {	6. Apical
	7. —
	8. Anterior basal
	9. Lateral basal
	10. Posterior basal

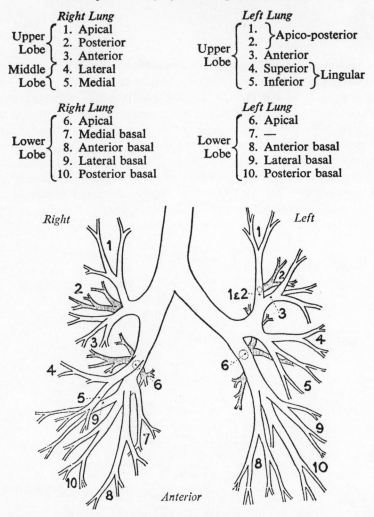

Fig. 1/4. Diagram illustrating the bronchopulmonary nomenclature approved by the Thoracic Society. (Reproduced by permission of the Editors of *Thorax*)

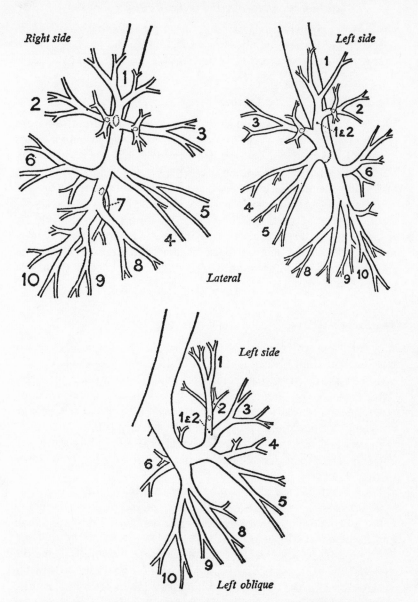

FIG. 1/4. Diagram illustrating the bronchopulmonary nomenclature approved by the Thoracic Society. (Reproduced by permission of the Editors of *Thorax*)

vocal cords extend between them and the angle of the thyroid cartilage.

The epiglottis lies just above the vocal cords and is shaped like a leaf. It may serve to direct food and liquids into the oesophagus.

The Trachea

The trachea is a tube about 12 cm long extending from the cricoid cartilage of the larynx (C.6) to the sternal angle (T.5) where it bifurcates to form the right and left main bronchi. It passes down in an oblique direction, its upper end in the neck being just below the skin and its lower end being adjacent to the vertebral column in the thorax. The framework of the trachea is provided by sixteen to twenty C-shaped pieces of cartilage. The circle is completed posteriorly by smooth involuntary muscle and the cartilages are joined together by fibro-elastic tissue. The cartilage at the bifurcation is shaped to support it and the bifurcation is frequently referred to as the carina (see Fig. 1/3).

The Bronchial Tree

The cartilages of the main bronchi are in the form of irregular plaques. The right bronchus is wider and shorter than the left and is nearly vertical in direction, being only slightly deviated to the right. After entering the lung at the hilum it divides into three branches, one for each of the three lobes. The left main bronchus is longer than the right and is directed more obliquely, passing below the arch of the aorta and in front of the oesophagus and descending aorta. On entering the lung at the hilum it divides into two to supply the lobes of the left lung.

Each lobar branch divides into segmental bronchi and each segmental bronchus together with the part of the lung it supplies is called a bronchopulmonary segment. The segments have both names and numbers (see Figs. 1/4 and 1/5).

These segments can be identified on the surface of the lung and the direction of each segmental bronchus is known although there are variations from the norm. This knowledge is the basis for postural drainage of the lungs, see Chapter 5, page 113.

It will be noted that the segments are named according to their position but it should always be borne in mind that the lung is divided by an oblique fissure. Thus the apex of the lower lobe

Outline of Anatomy of the Respiratory System

reaches as high as T.3 and lies posterior to but on a level with the posterior and anterior segments of the upper lobe.

Branching of the bronchial tree continues and the diameter of the lumen decreases until at about 0·2 mm the tube is known as a bronchiole. Still further branching takes place until the terminal bronchioles are reached. The bronchial tree down to this level has relatively thick walls containing irregular plates of hyaline cartilage. It is lined by ciliated epithelium. The main control of the airway diameter is exerted by circular muscle fibres in the smaller and terminal bronchioles. The bronchioles are prevented from collapsing by the radial traction of the adjacent lung tissue.

The terminal bronchiole is followed by a thin-walled tube, the respiratory bronchiole (see Fig. 1/6).

Alveoli

Leading from the respiratory bronchiole are the alveolar ducts. Each one opens into a large central area, the alveolar sac, around the periphery of which lie the alveoli or air saccules. The cavities are lined with simple flat epithelium which is in contact with the pulmonary capillary network. At this level gaseous exchange takes place.

COLLATERAL AIR DRIFT
Air can pass between adjacent alveoli through the pores of Kohn unless they are separated by septa, and Lambert has described accessory communications between some bronchioles and adjacent alveoli. This passage of air is called collateral ventilation or collateral air drift.

Blood Supply

The bronchial arteries which are branches of the aorta supply the bronchial tree itself and the visceral pleura. The bronchial veins drain into the azygos system.

The pulmonary arteries convey deoxygenated blood to the lungs from the right ventricle and the pulmonary veins (two for each lung) convey oxygenated blood from the capillary network to the left atrium of the heart.

29

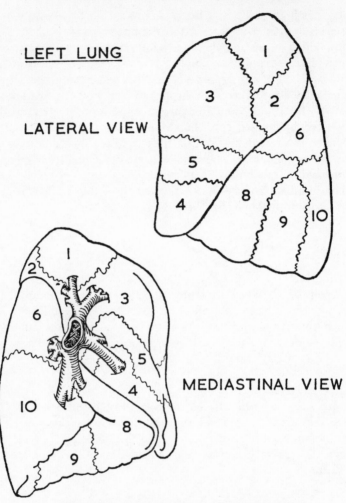

FIG. 1/5 (a). Left bronchopulmonary segments

Nerve Supply

The nerve supply is provided by the autonomic system.

30

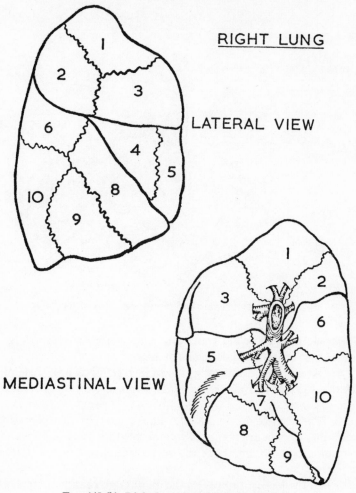

RIGHT LUNG

LATERAL VIEW

MEDIASTINAL VIEW

FIG. 1/5 (b). Right bronchopulmonary segments

MECHANISM OF RESPIRATION

Inspiration

IN QUIET INSPIRATION
1. The thoracic inlet remains at rest.
2. The second to seventh true ribs rotate in two directions:
a) About the sternovertebral axis. This is called the 'bucket

31

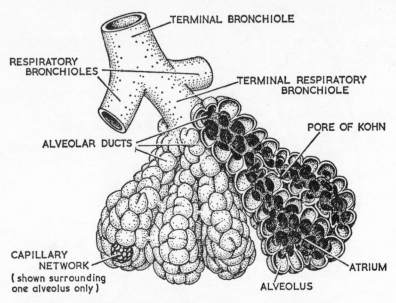

FIG. 1/6. The conducting and respiratory parts of the lungs

handle' action. Thus the transverse diameter of the thorax is increased and the subcostal angle widened.

b) About the costovertebral joint in a 'pump handle' fashion so that the anterior end moves upwards increasing the anteroposterior thoracic diameter.

3. The muscle fibres of the diaphragm contract. The upper abdominal viscera are compressed and the abdominal muscles relax to accommodate them. Thus the vertical diameter of the thorax is increased.

On slightly deeper inspiration the diaphragm cannot compress the viscera further and the central tendon becomes the fixed point at the level of T.9. Further contraction of the diaphragmatic muscle fibres causes the lower ribs to rise and the body of the sternum to move forwards. Some authorities doubt this and think that this is probably an integrated activity no matter what degree of diaphragmatic contraction occurs.

As can be seen in Fig. 1/7, when the diaphragm contracts A tends to move up because of rib anatomy. This widens the thorax. Simultaneously B moves down and increases the vertical diameter.

IN DEEP INSPIRATION

The scalene muscles and the sternal head of sternomastoid come into action to raise the first and second ribs, and all the intercostal muscles which aid inspiration are brought into action.

FORCED INSPIRATION

This occurs during periods of respiratory distress. Inspiration is

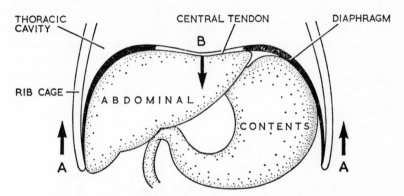

FIG. 1/7. Diagram illustrating diaphragmatic contraction

increased by the use of pectoralis minor and perhaps pectoralis major and serratus anterior which can be brought into action by fixing the scapula. This is usually done by fixing the whole of the upper limb by gripping something suitably stable, for example a table.

Trapezius, levator scapulae and the rhomboids may also take part if the head and neck are fixed by the necessary muscles.

The scaleni and the sternal head of sternomastoid together with the muscles mentioned under Forced Inspiration are referred to as accessory muscles of respiration.

Expiration

Normal quiet expiration is due to the elastic recoil of the tissues. Forced expiration is brought about by contraction of the abdominal muscles and latissimus dorsi and in extreme cases by pressure of the arms upon the chest wall.

Coughing

This is a reflex action brought about by stimulation of the sensory nerves present in the larynx or trachea. It may also be caused by stimulation of the afferent nerve endings in the lungs or pleura. All these afferent nerve endings are supplied by the vagus nerve. A short but deep inspiration is followed by closure of the vocal cords. There is a forced expiratory effort which, because of the closed larynx, results in a build-up of high pressure within the lungs and bronchial tree. Suddenly, the vocal cords open and the air thus released escapes with an explosive force carrying with it anything lying in the respiratory passages. Sometimes the air flows at a rate of 70 miles per hour.

Sneezing is a similar mechanism and is caused by irritation of the membranes of the nose. Variations in the position of the soft palate allow the rapid flow of air through the nose and mouth, clearing the nasal pathways.

SURFACE MARKING

Larynx

Third cervical vertebra to lower border of sixth cervical vertebra.

Trachea

Sixth cervical vertebra to sternal angle or fourth to fifth thoracic vertebra. (The sternum articulates with the second costal cartilage at the sternal angle.)

Pleura

Apex 3 cm (approx.) above the clavicle beneath the clavicular head of sternomastoid.

A line joining the following points gives the outline.

1. Sternoclavicular joint.

2. Right and left converge to the sternal angle and meet just to the left of mid-line.

3. Vertically down to the level of the fourth chondrosternal junction.

4. Right continues obliquely to the sixth or seventh chondrosternal junction.

Left passes outwards and downwards behind the costal cartilages of fifth, sixth, seventh and eighth ribs.

5. Both right and left pass laterally

    a) eighth costal cartilage—lateral vertical line.

    b) tenth rib   —mid-axillary line.

    c) eleventh rib   —in line with inferior angle of scapula.

    d) twelfth vertebrocostal joint.

6. Otherwise the pleura follows the walls of the thoracic cavity.

Lungs

1. Root—Posterior aspect of the thorax at the level of the fifth and sixth ribs halfway between the medial border of the scapula and the spinous processes.

2. Apex—Above the clavicle beneath the clavicular head of sternomastoid.

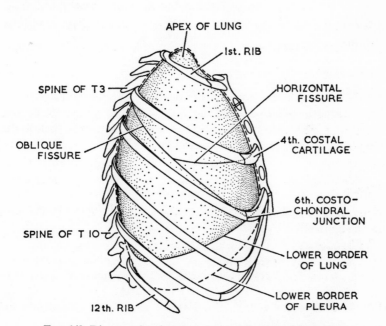

Fig. 1/8. Diagram showing the lobes and fissures of the lungs and pleura related to the thoracic cage

35

3. Sternal angle.
4. Right lung. A line joining the following points.

a) passes vertically down to the sixth or seventh chondro-sternal junction.

    b) sixth costal cartilage—lateral vertical line.

    c) eighth rib   —mid-axillary line.

    d) tenth rib   —line of inferior angle of scapula.

    e) tenth thoracic spine.

5. Left lung. A line joining the following points.

a) lies behind the left border of the sternum to the fourth chondrosternal junction.

    b) passes outwards along the fourth costal cartilage.

    c) curves down to the sixth costal cartilage.

    d) follows line described for the right lung.

6. Fissures—Oblique fissure on the right and left from the spine of the third thoracic vertebra posteriorly to the sixth costochondral junction anteriorly.

—Horizontal fissure on the right from the oblique fissure in the mid-axillary line to the fourth costal cartilage anteriorly (see Fig. 1/8).

Diaphragm

Levels vary with the position of the body. The diaphragm takes origin from the margins of the thoracic outlet and rises to the central tendon on each side of which it has a rounded cupola below the lungs and is depressed slightly in the middle.

	Anterior	Posterior
Median Portion	Xiphisternal joint	Body T.9. Spine T.8
Right Cupola	fifth rib 1–2 cm below right nipple	1–2 cm below inferior angle of scapula
	Anterior	Posterior
Left Cupola	fifth interspace or sixth rib 2·5 cm below left nipple	2·5 cm below the inferior angle of scapula

Chest Measurement Levels

1. Fourth costal cartilage.
2. Xiphoid process.
3. Ninth costal cartilage (anterior extremity).

REFERENCES AND BIBLIOGRAPHY

Best, C. H. & Taylor, N. B. (1959). *The Living Body*. Chapman & Hall Ltd., London. 4th ed.

Cotes, J. E. (1968). *Lung Function—Assessment and Application in Medicine*. Blackwell Scientific Publications, Oxford. 2nd ed.

Grant, J. C. B. (1971). *A Method of Anatomy*. Churchill-Livingstone, Edinburgh. 8th ed.

Gray's Anatomy—Illustrated and Applied. 35th ed. 1973 (edited by R. Warwick), Longman Group Ltd., London.

Hamilton, W. J. & Simon, G. (1971). *Surface and Radiological Anatomy*. W. Heffer & Sons Ltd., Cambridge. 5th ed.

Last, R. J. (1972). *Anatomy—Regional and Applied*. Churchill-Livingstone, Edinburgh. 5th ed.

Mitchell, G. A. G. & Patterson, E. L. (1967). *Basic Anatomy*. Churchill-Livingstone, Edinburgh. 2nd ed.

Passmore, R. & Robinson, J. S. (1971) (Eds in Chief). *A Companion to Medical Studies*. Vol. 1. Blackwell Scientific Publications, Oxford. 3rd ed.

Rawling's Landmarks and Surface Markings. 9th ed. 1953 (revised by Robinson, J. O.). H. K. Lewis & Co. Ltd., London.

CHAPTER 2

The Basic Physiology of Respiration

by P. J. WADDINGTON, M.C.S.P., H.T., DIP.T.P.

Purpose of Respiration

Breathing is the first and last act of the respiratory process which is concerned with the intake of oxygen and the elimination of carbon dioxide by the body. Respiration is also concerned with the regulation of the hydrogen ion concentration of the blood.

The process involves:

1. Ventilation—the mass movement of air in and out of the lungs.

2. The exchange of oxygen and carbon dioxide between the alveolar air and the pulmonary capillaries.

3. Blood gas transport to and from the tissues.

4. Gaseous exchange at tissue level.

Act of Breathing

INSPIRATION

This is an active muscular effort designed to enlarge the thoracic cavity, lowering the intrathoracic pressure to a subatmospheric level. As this occurs air flows from a region of higher pressure (atmospheric) to one of lower pressure (subatmospheric).

The inspiratory effort has the following forces to overcome.

1. External forces.

2. Elastic recoil of the lungs and thorax.

3. Frictional resistance to the movement of the tissues.

4. The resistance to airflow by the bronchial tree itself.

38

EXPIRATION

Normal quiet expiration is caused by the elastic recoil of the tissues. If the resistance given to the moving gases by the non-elastic tissues of the airway is negligible, the return of the lungs to their resting position is quick and easy but where resistance is above normal, the speed of expiration will be reduced and active contraction of the expiratory muscles may be necessary. The expiratory muscles will be contracted during forced expiratory acts such as blowing and coughing etc.

ELASTICITY AND COMPLIANCE

Both the lungs and the thoracic cage contain tissues which have elastic properties. Elasticity of a body is defined as the property of a body to return to its original shape after it has been distorted by some external force. These structures obey Hook's Law—'Stress is proportional to strain' or 'Equal increases in a force cause equal increases in length'. The force is provided by the muscles of inspiration. The work in changing the original shape of the body is stored as potential energy which is expended as the body returns to normal. The reciprocal of elasticity is compliance, which is a measure of the distensibility of the lung. In many patients with lung disease compliance is reduced whilst in some, for example, those with emphysema, it may be increased.

Elastic Forces Acting Upon Lungs and Thorax

In the normal subject who is relaxed at the end of quiet expiration the elastic forces of the lungs and thorax balance one another. That is, the tendency of the elasticity of the lungs to empty them is equal to the tendency of the elastic forces of the thorax to expand. If air enters between the pleura of the lung and chest wall, the lung will collapse and the chest wall will move outwards. In conditions such as emphysema where the elasticity of the lung is lost, the unopposed elasticity of the thorax causes it to expand. The elastic forces of the thorax have a limit giving the thorax a fixed capacity which will vary with the individual. Therefore rigidity of the thorax in disease will have an adverse effect on respiration.

Lung elasticity is not solely dependent upon collagenous and

39

elastic fibres but also upon the fact that a surface tension exists between the liquid lining the alveoli and the alveolar gas. This force tends to cause the alveolus to collapse. Therefore the inspiratory muscles must overcome this alveolar surface tension as well as tissue elasticity when they inflate the lungs.

Frictional Resistance to Respiration

There are two types:

1. The friction caused by the movement of the tissues, that is, the rib-cage, diaphragm, abdominal structures and the lungs themselves during inspiration and expiration.

2. The friction caused during the flow of gases, a) between the molecules of the gases themselves, b) between the gases and the walls of the tubes.

During slow flow in a straight tube the flow is laminar, that is, in straight lines like the laminae of a piece of plywood seen from the side. The air in the centre of the tube flows faster than that at the periphery.

During fast flow in a straight tube the air flowing along becomes turbulent.

Because of the many branching tubes in the bronchial tree, eddy currents are set up which may create turbulence even at moderate flow rates.

The effect of abnormalities in the smooth tubes of the bronchial tree which may be caused by excessive mucus secretions or tumours is to increase the turbulence of the gases passing through.

LUNG VOLUMES

All lung volumes are related to the physique of the subject.

The volume of air that can be expelled from the lungs following the deepest possible inspiration is called the *vital capacity* (V.C.). The average man will have a V.C. of about 4·5 litres and the average woman 3·2 litres (see Fig. 2/1).

In normal quiet respiration we neither breathe in fully nor out fully. Therefore we have an *inspiratory reserve volume* (I.R.V.) and an *expiratory reserve volume* (E.R.V.) in addition to the air passing in and out during quiet respiration which is called *tidal volume* (T.V.).

$$\left.\begin{array}{l}\text{I.R.V.} = 2\cdot6 \text{ litres}\\ \text{E.R.V.} = 1\cdot5 \text{ litres}\\ \text{T.V.} = 0\cdot4 \text{ litres}\end{array}\right\} = \text{V.C. } 4\cdot5 \text{ litres}$$
(calculated on a total
lung capacity of 6 litres)

At the end of quiet expiration, that is, at the *resting respiratory level*, 3·0 litres of air remains in the lungs. This is called the *functional residual capacity* (F.R.C.). It is composed of the E.R.V. = 1·5 litres and the *residual volume* (R.V.) which is 1·5 litres and cannot be forced out of the lungs, remaining in the alveoli.

$$\left.\begin{array}{l}\text{E.R.V.} = 1\cdot5 \text{ litres}\\ \text{R.V.} = 1\cdot5 \text{ litres}\end{array}\right\} = \text{F.R.C. } 3\cdot0 \text{ litres}$$
(calculated on a total
lung capacity of 6 litres)

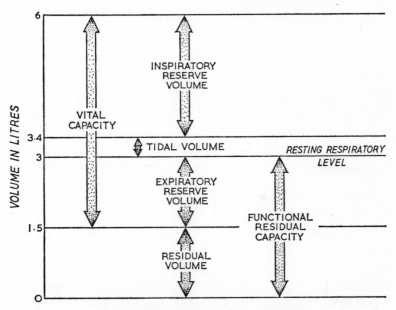

FIG. 2/1. Diagram showing lung volumes

Forced Expiratory Volume

It is usual to measure V.C. with a spirometer, to give an indication of the condition of the patient's lungs. This is most often made using a dry, waterless spirometer, the Vitalograph. If the vital capacity is forced out as rapidly and completely as possible it is called the *forced expiratory volume* (F.E.V.). A most significant figure in

41

assessing a patient is the F.E.V. which occurs in the first second, the F.E.V.$_1$. In a normal person this is usually at least 70% of the total V.C. In patients with diffuse airways obstruction this percentage is considerably reduced. The Vitalograph apparatus produces a permanent record in the form of a graph which may be kept in the patient's notes.

Maximal Ventilation Volume

Another measurement of lung function which is considered to be of clinical value is the *maximal ventilation volume* or the *maximal voluntary ventilation* (M.V.V.). The subject is asked to breathe as deeply and rapidly as possible for 15 seconds and the ventilation per minute is then calculated. In normal subjects the volume may be greater than 100 litres per minute.

Peak Flow

Peak flow is another lung function test. In this the patient's highest expiratory flow rate during forced expiration is measured. This test is related to F.E.V.$_1$ and M.V.V.

Rate of Respiration

The rate of respiration is about 14 breaths per minute for normal subjects at rest.

Dead Space

The tidal volume passing in and out of the lungs during normal quiet respiration equals about 400 ml; of this only 250 ml reaches the alveoli. The remaining 150 ml is still in the air passages at the end of inspiration and can therefore take no part in gaseous exchange. Therefore the volume of each breath must exceed 150 ml. Below this level breathing will not be useful. This 150 ml is called *anatomical dead space*. In patients with a tracheostomy this is decreased.

The air which enters the alveoli is called alveolar air. Of this some may not be used to oxygenate the blood flowing through pulmonary capillaries because too much enters the alveoli in proportion to their blood flow. In some patients a proportion of the alveoli may have no

42

blood flow at all and the air which reaches these cannot be utilised, so that the air passing to and fro serves no respiratory function. The volume of inspired air which enters the alveoli and is of no functional value is also effectively 'dead space' gas. Alveolar dead space plus anatomical dead space is usually called physiological dead space.

Percentage of Gases

	Inspired Air %	Alveolar Air %	Expired Air %
O_2	21	14	16
CO_2	0	6	4
N_2	79	80	80

Air in the alveoli in quiet respiration will be a mixture of the lungs' functional residual capacity and 250 ml of the tidal volume. Therefore it will be of a lower oxygen and a higher carbon dioxide content than room air. Expired air will have a higher oxygen and a lower carbon dioxide content than alveolar air because it is a mixture of alveolar air and dead space air which will contain room air percentage of gases.

This larger percentage of oxygen in expired air than in alveolar air is a vital statistic when mouth-to-mouth breathing is being given.

CARRIAGE OF GASES—PARTIAL PRESSURES

The air in the respiratory system is composed of a mixture of three gases and water vapour. The proportions of oxygen and carbon dioxide are variable while that of nitrogen remains the same.

The physical properties of this mixture can be deduced from:

DALTON'S LAWS OF PARTIAL PRESSURES

1. 'The pressure exerted by a mixture of gases is equal to the sum of the pressures which each would exert if it alone occupied the space.'

2. 'The pressure exerted by a saturated vapour depends only upon the temperature and the particular liquid considered.'

BOYLE'S LAW

'The volume of a fixed mass of gas is inversely proportional to the pressure provided the temperature is constant.'

The Basic Physiology of Respiration

It follows, therefore, that the partial pressure of any gas is proportional to its percentage by volume in the mixture.

Therefore when three gases, oxygen, carbon dioxide and nitrogen occupy the same space, each will contribute to the total pressure in proportion to its concentration. The actual pressure measured in millimetres of mercury will vary with the barometric pressure.

It must be remembered that alveolar air is saturated with water vapour at body temperature. At 37° C water vapour in alveolar air has a pressure of 47 mm Hg independent of the gases and not variable with barometric pressure.

PARTIAL PRESSURES IN ALVEOLAR AIR

$$O_2 = 14\% \text{ of } 760\text{—}47 \text{ mm Hg} = 100 \text{ mm Hg}$$
$$CO_2 = 6\% \text{ of } 760\text{—}47 \text{ mm Hg} = 40 \text{ mm Hg}$$

That is $PO_2 = 100$ and the $PCO_2 = 40$

HENRY'S LAW OF SOLUTION

'The quantity of gas going into a simple solution at constant temperature is proportional to the pressure.' *Dalton states* that

'In a mixture of gases the solubility of each gas varies proportionally with its partial pressure.'

Therefore the movement of gases between a gas and a liquid or between liquids is governed by pressures. The movement is always from one of high pressure to one of low pressure. The movement of gases in the lungs between the alveolar air and the blood, is in a gas to liquid situation, oxygen moving into the blood and carbon dioxide into the air. At tissue level, a liquid to liquid situation, oxygen moves into the tissues and carbon dioxide from the tissues into the blood.

PARTIAL PRESSURES

In alveolar air and arterial blood PO_2 is 100 mm Hg approx
In alveolar air and arterial blood PCO_2 is 40 mm Hg approx
In tissues and venous blood PO_2 is 40 mm Hg approx
In tissues and venous blood PCO_2 is 46 mm Hg approx

Gases are carried in the blood as a result of:
1. The formation of a solution.
2. Chemical combination.

The amount carried is dependent upon tension or partial pressure.

Carriage of Oxygen

IN SOLUTION—DISSOLVED IN PLASMA
A small volume of oxygen, which can be calculated to be 0·3 vols. per cent, is carried in the blood in solution. It is of little significance when oxygen supply to the tissues is being considered.

CHEMICAL COMBINATION—COMBINED WITH HAEMOGLOBIN
The amount of oxygen combined with haemoglobin in a red cell is dependent upon oxygen tension or pressure and can be represented on a graph as an S-shaped curve, the *oxygen dissociation curve* (see Fig. 2/2). When the PO_2 equals 100 the haemoglobin of the red cells is 97·4% saturated. This is called the *arterial point*. Because the haemoglobin is nearly 100% saturated at this point the graph is plotted as PO_2 against percentage saturation of haemoglobin. At a PO_2 of 40 the haemoglobin is 70% saturated. This is called the *venous point*.

The quantity of oxygen which the blood is able to carry is dependent upon:

1. The amount of haemoglobin in the red cells.

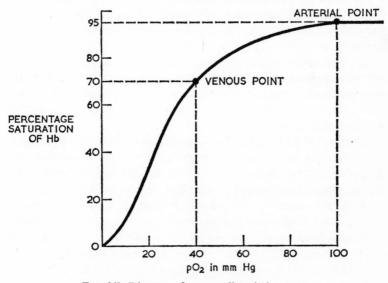

FIG. 2/2. Diagram of oxygen dissociation curve

45

2. The number of red cells.

3. The amount of carbon dioxide carried by the blood.

If the PCO_2 is raised less oxygen is carried at a given tension.

The PO_2 of blood as it passes through the lungs is raised from 40 mm Hg to 100 mm Hg. This represents 5 ml of oxygen for every 100 ml of blood.

Carriage of Carbon Dioxide

IN SOLUTION

Some carbon dioxide dissolves in the plasma and a small quantity of this reacts with water to form carbonic acid. As carbonic acid is a weak acid very few of its molecules dissociate into H^+ and HCO_3^-

$$H_2O + CO_2 \rightleftharpoons H_2CO_3 \rightleftharpoons H^+ + HCO_3^-$$

In addition, some carbon dioxide dissolves within the erythrocytes.

CHEMICAL COMBINATION

1. Carbon dioxide combines with the amino group of plasma proteins to form carbamino compounds.

2. Carbon dioxide also combines with the amine (NH_2^-) part of the haemoglobin molecule. Oxygen combines with the iron (haem) radical. Saturation of haemoglobin with carbon dioxide occurs at a low partial pressure and the reaction is very speedy, requiring no catalyst.

3. Formation of bicarbonate. Carbon dioxide from the tissues enters the plasma and diffuses quickly across the cell membrane into the erythrocyte. Because of the presence within the red cells of the catalyst carbonic anhydrase, the reaction $H_2O + CO_2 \rightleftharpoons H_2CO_3$ is accelerated.

Reduced haemoglobin which results from the release of oxygen to the tissues acts as a base and mops up the H^+ released from the $H_2CO_3 \rightleftharpoons H^+ + HCO_3^-$. The HCO_3^- thus liberated diffuses out of the red cell and is replaced by Cl^- from the plasma. This maintains the ionic balance across the cell membrane and is called the *chloride shift*. Within the red cells the Cl^- combines with K^+ forming potassium chloride and in the plasma HCO_3^- combines with Na^+ to form sodium bicarbonate.

In the lungs the haemoglobin becomes oxygenated and the process is reversed.

Carbon dioxide dissociation curves of blood and plasma can be plotted (see Fig. 2/3). But full saturation of the blood by carbon dioxide does not occur. Therefore they are not plotted in the same way as the oxygen dissociation curve, that is, as percentages of saturation. They are plotted as partial pressures against volumes per cent. Over the normal range of PCO_2 there is only a slight curve so that it nearly represents a straight line.

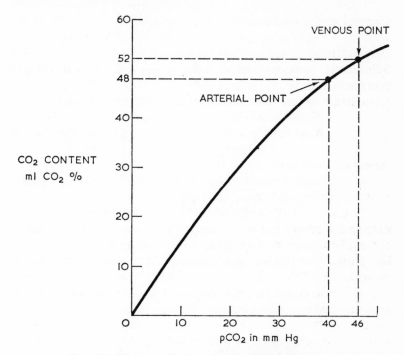

FIG. 2/3. Diagram of carbon dioxide dissociation curve

Maintenance of Blood pH

In health the pH of the blood is maintained within very narrow limits, *i.e.* 7·35–7·45. This is a slightly alkaline solution. The acidity or alkalinity of a solution is dependent upon the concentrations of hydrogen ions H^+ and hydroxyl ions OH^-. The use of the pH method is a way of expressing this and is sometimes referred to as the hydrogen ion concentration, to which it is inversely related. pH 7 indicates a neutral solution. Any figure below seven shows acidity, *i.e.* an increase in hydrogen ion concentration, any figure above seven indicates a decrease in the hydrogen ion concentration and therefore an alkaline solution.

The pH of whole blood or plasma depends upon the ratio of the bicarbonate and carbonic acid present. The blood bicarbonate is an important chemical buffer in the regulation of acid-base balance.

Carbon dioxide from the tissues is constantly entering the blood and combining with water to form carbonic acid. Under normal conditions an equal amount of carbon dioxide is expelled by the lungs and the pH of the blood is not affected. If this elimination of carbon dioxide is reduced the carbonic acid content of the blood will rise. This increase in acid will cause the pH to fall. A reduction in pH is referred to as acidosis.

If there is an increase in the ventilation of the lungs and carbon dioxide is expelled at above the normal rate the CO_2 and H_2CO_3 concentration in the blood will fall, it will become more alkaline and the pH will rise, *i.e.* a proportionate rise in bicarbonate will cause a rise in the pH. This is called alkalosis.

CONTROL OF RESPIRATION

Respiration is an involuntary activity which to a certain extent is under voluntary control. One can stop breathing and control its rate and depth but breathing cannot be stopped for an indefinite period; approximately 45 seconds is the maximum. Breathing is also modified at an involuntary level during such activities as speaking, swallowing and coughing etc.

Nervous Control of Respiration

Spontaneous respiration is due to a rhythmic electrical discharge from a group of nerve cells in the reticular formation of the brain stem, mainly in the lower part of the floor of the fourth ventricle in the medulla. This area is called the *respiratory centre*. Some cells form the *expiratory centre* and are situated more posteriorly than the group of cells forming the *inspiratory centre* but their territories overlap. Although this area has been designated as the respiratory centre, it is now thought that for normal respiration it is necessary for the whole of the reticular formation to be functioning. Damage to the respiratory centre is in many cases fatal.

From this area impulses are sent to C.3, 4 and 5 for relay to the diaphragm via the phrenic nerve and to the thoracic spinal cord for relay by the intercostal nerves to supply the intercostal muscles, the diaphragm and the abdominal muscles.

The exact way in which the neurones of the reticular formation interrelate has yet to be established but from this area rhythmic inspiratory and expiratory impulses are discharged. These can be influenced by afferent impulses reaching the area.

THE HERING-BREUER REFLEX

Many vagal afferent fibres are present in the walls of the small air passages. They are sensitive to stretch. When the lungs are inflated, impulses are generated which have an inhibitory effect on the inspiratory centre. The greater the stretch the greater the inhibition.

When the lungs are deflated for a prolonged period there is an increase in inspiratory effort. Again it is considered that afferent impulses are conveyed along vagal afferent fibres.

Some authorities consider that both these reflexes form the Hering-Breuer reflex. In man the Hering-Breuer reflex is very weak.

COUGH REFLEX

The vagus nerve probably carries the afferent impulses initiated by the irritants which stimulate a cough reflex. The upper part of the respiratory tract is sensitive to mechanical irritants while the alveoli are sensitive to chemical substances.

PRESSURE

The carotid sinuses and carotid bodies are affected by pressure and are called baroreceptors. When they are stimulated by a rise in blood pressure this has an inhibitory effect on the respiratory centre. A fall in blood pressure has the opposite effect.

CHEMORECEPTORS

The carotid bodies which lie one on each side of the carotid bifurcation and the aortic bodies which lie near the arch of the aorta are sensitive to oxygen lack. Their afferent impulses pass along the glossopharyngeal and vagus nerves respectively and share the same nerve trunk as the afferents of the baroreceptors. They have a stimulating effect on the respiratory centre. N.B. The direct effect of anoxia on the respiratory centre is depressing.

49

Stimulation of the respiratory centre by oxygen lack is not a very important factor under normal conditions, as haemoglobin is easily saturated with oxygen at normal or even below normal rates of ventilation. However, it is important at high altitudes where the oxygen concentration in the atmosphere is low, resulting in inadequate oxygenation of haemoglobin.

In some respiratory diseases the patients may 'learn' to tolerate high carbon dioxide levels in the blood. Stimulation of the respiratory centre by oxygen lack can then become a vital factor.

In these cases it can be dangerous to give the patient too much oxygen as this stimulation to respiration will thus have been removed.

OTHER INFLUENCES

A change in body temperature, especially a sudden cooling, for example if one were to jump into the sea on Christmas Day, will cause hyperventilation.

It is thought that the proprioceptors present in the muscles of respiration may influence the respiratory centre.

The respiratory rate is influenced by higher centres and changes in rate, depth and rhythm are brought about by emotional factors.

The respiratory centre is depressed during sleep causing an increase in alveolar carbon dioxide.

Chemical Control of Breathing

CARBON DIOXIDE

It is a matter for debate whether the PCO_2 or the hydrogen ion concentration of the blood is the most important single factor to stimulate the respiratory centre producing both an increase in the rate and depth of respiration.

If the air in the alveoli has a high PCO_2 the arterial blood being in equilibrium with it will also have a high PCO_2. This high level of carbon dioxide will increase ventilation by directly affecting the respiratory centre.

An increase of carbon dioxide in the blood is reflected in a rise of carbon dioxide, in the form of carbonic acid, in the cerebrospinal fluid. The rise in the hydrogen ion concentration thus effected has an excitatory influence on the respiratory centre which lies in the floor of the fourth ventricle.

The blood pH is kept constant by the balance of bicarbonate and carbonic acid. The kidneys regulate the bicarbonate concentration of the plasma despite variation in the dietary intake. An increase in the amount of carbonic acid, due to a rise in the carbon dioxide in the blood, will be reflected in an increase in the hydrogen ion concentration. This is represented by a fall in pH. A fall in the pH of the blood has an excitatory effect on the respiratory centre. (Release of acids other than carbonic, *e.g.* lactic acid from exercising muscle or ketoacids in diabetes will stimulate breathing in a similar way.)

It must be remembered that PCO_2 and pH are interrelated as the amount of carbon dioxide in solution in the blood is dependent upon carbon dioxide tension.

Very high concentrations of carbon dioxide in the blood have a narcotic effect and can lead to unconsciousness and death.

OXYGEN TENSION

Oxygen lack as given above is registered by the chemoreceptors which influence the respiratory centre via afferent nerve impulses. This therefore can be classified as nervous control.

The direct effect (chemical) of oxygen lack on the respiratory centre is depressing.

TABLE OF NORMAL VALUES

Lung Volumes based on a Capacity of 6 litres
Vital Capacity (V.C.)   = 4·5 litres
Residual Volume (R.V.)   = 1·5 litres
Expiratory Reserve Volume (E.R.V.) = 1·5 litres
Functional Residual Capacity (F.R.C.) = 3·0 litres
Tidal Volume (T.V.)   = 0·4 litres
                                (400 ml)
Inspiratory Reserve Volume (I.R.V.) = 2·6 litres
Forced Expiratory Volume in the 1st Second (F.E.V.₁) = 70% V.C.
Maximum Ventilation Volume (M.V.V.) = 100 litres
Anatomical Dead Space   = 150 ml

Partial Pressures
Alveolar Air and Arterial Blood $PO_2 = 100$ mm Hg; $PCO_2 = 40$ mm Hg
Tissues and Venous Blood $PO_2 = 40$ mm Hg; $PCO_2 = 46$ mm Hg
Blood pH $= 7·4$ (slightly alkaline)
Vital capacity of the average male = 4·5 litres approx
                     female = 3·2 litres approx
Rate of Respiration 14–20 per minute

REFERENCES AND BIBLIOGRAPHY

Comroe, J. H., Forster, R. E., Dubois, A. B., Briscoe, W. A. & Carlson, Eliza-
beth (1970). *The Lung: Clinical Physiology and Pulmonary Function Tests.*
Year Book Medical Publishers Inc., Chicago.

Green, J. H. (1968). *An Introduction to Human Physiology.* Oxford University
Press. 2nd ed.

Guyton, A. C. (1969). *Function of the Human Body.* W. B. Saunders Co. 3rd ed.

Passmore, R. & Robson, J. S. (1971) (Eds in Chief). *A Companion to Medical
Studies.* Blackwell Scientific Publications, Oxford. 3rd ed.

CHAPTER 3

Intensive Care—1

by P. J. WADDINGTON, M.C.S.P., H.T., DIP.T.P.

What is Intensive Care?

Progressive patient care has always been a feature of hospital life. In the traditional type of ward, patients who require constant care and supervision are placed in beds near to the Sister's office where they are always under the watchful eye of the staff passing to and fro. As the condition of the patient improves he is moved farther down the ward where the supervision based on simple geography will be less.

With the development of more sophisticated equipment and techniques the commissioning of *intensive care units* became a natural development of the graduated ward method. Such units ensure the best and most economical use of personnel and equipment.

In large hospitals it is usual to have several units where specialized patient care is given, for example a respiratory care unit, a cardiac surgery unit, a renal unit and a coronary care unit. Intensive care and supervision of patients is given on all these units and yet it is unusual for a physiotherapist to be asked to treat someone in a coronary care unit, and her services are only required spasmodically on the renal unit. The question therefore may be asked: 'What do we mean by intensive care?' Many patients receive intensive physiotherapy, for example, in a thoracic surgery ward or rehabilitation centre, but this is not usually classified as intensive care.

Here intensive care includes patients who, without mechanical aid in some form, even if this is only suction, would be unable to maintain adequate ventilation; that is intensive respiratory care. The majority of these patients will be nursed on a specialized unit with

53

well-trained staff, others will be scattered throughout the hospital where, perhaps, only the senior nursing staff will have received the necessary training.

Conditions from which these patients suffer vary and can include, for example, the patient who may be unconscious following a cerebrovascular accident or a head injury, one who has returned from the theatre after a heart valve replacement, another who is completely paralysed with polyneuritis and yet another with diffuse obstructive disease of the airways who requires intensive care to help him through an acute exacerbation of his condition.

The essence of effective intensive care is teamwork and, as in any good team, the members have certain basic skills and knowledge in common but it is the blending of different talents which together make an effective whole. Everyone has one simple objective, the recovery of the patient. The personnel of the unit will include the physician or surgeon, the anaesthetist, nursing staff, the technicians who maintain the equipment and the physiotherapists. The services of the radiographers and the laboratory technicians are regularly required. In some units either the physician or surgeon will be in charge, in others the anaesthetist.

It is obvious that intensive care is a service which must be available 24 hours a day, seven days a week, including Christmas Day and Boxing Day. This is not to say that a physiotherapist has always to be on duty all night. In many cases this is not necessary; usually if the patient has been treated at regular intervals during the day and again in the evening he can be safely left at night. He needs his sleep too. However, an 'on call' service must be arranged.

HISTORY

Modern intensive respiratory care is a development of the work of a Danish doctor, Dr. H. C. A. Lassen and an anaesthetist, Dr. B. Ibsen who, in the poliomyelitis epidemic in 1952, were faced with the problem of treating patients who could not swallow or breathe, which with the equipment available at that time was a fatal combination.

The first co-ordinated records of attempts to design breathing machines appear to be associated with the founding of the Humane Society (later the Royal Humane Society) in 1774. In relatively modern times (1929) a practical breathing machine was designed by

Dr. Phillip Drinker, an engineer of Harvard University. This respirator and its successors, were based on the *negative (subatmospheric) pressure principle*. It was called the 'iron lung' by the general public; the correct name of this type of respirator is the *tank* or *cabinet respirator.*

The tank respirator was an air-tight box designed to take the whole of the patient's body and limbs, leaving the head outside. Ways had to be found to ensure a good seal round the neck. In the original tanks the patient was placed on a drawer on wheels which could be pulled out from inside the cabinet. An improved model, the Smith-Clarke Cabinet Respirator, Alligator Model was produced in 1952. As the name implies, the lid of the respirator was hinged at the foot end and it opened rather like the jaws of an alligator. This was quick and easy to operate when the patient could not be cared for through the portholes which were placed at intervals along each side. It also had a face mask or mouthpiece which the patient could use when the cabinet was open.

In normal respiration a muscular effort produces a gradual increase in the volume of the thorax, pressure is reduced to subatmospheric levels and air enters the lungs via the respiratory passages from the nose and mouth which are at atmospheric pressure. This reduced pressure in the thorax also aids venous return to the heart. Because the surface of the body is at atmospheric pressure there is a favourable pressure gradient between the blood in the peripheral veins and the right atrium.

The cabinet respirator was attached to bellows which created a negative (subatmospheric) pressure within the box. The patient's nose and mouth, outside the box, were at atmospheric pressure. Thus air flowed into the patient's lungs until the difference between the pressure within the tank and the pressure within the lungs was equal to the elasticity of the lungs and the chest wall. This was an effective method of ventilating the lungs but it had an adverse effect on venous return to the heart. The peripheral veins were within the box, thus they were at subatmospheric pressure too and therefore there was no advantageous pressure gradient to aid venous return. To counter this it was usual to introduce a positive pressure phase into the cycle, especially for patients who were in the respirator for a long period.

There is a vital flaw in this method of ventilation when it is used for patients who cannot swallow and maintain a clear airway.

Secretions from the mouth which could include vomit may be drawn into the patient's lungs as well as air. The patient then either drowns or his lungs are damaged by the secretions. In some centres especially in the United States of America a cuffed tracheostomy tube (a tube in the trachea which bypasses the upper respiratory tract and is designed to prevent secretions from there from entering the lungs) was used to overcome this problem. The method worked well but the patient in the tank was a very difficult nursing problem at best. A new method of ventilating patients who could not swallow was necessary. Today, except for a few old 'polio patients' who may sleep in the tank, it is very unlikely that a negative pressure respirator will be used; the positive pressure ventilator is a much more practical proposition even for the patient who can swallow.

The method instituted by Dr. Lassen was based on two ideas, the maintaining of a clear airway and the use of positive pressure ventilation, that is blowing air into the lungs, which at the beginning was provided by manual pressure on a rubber bag as used in anaesthetics. The manpower was provided by medical students working day and night on a rota basis. It was not long before a mechanical ventilator was designed to undertake this onerous task. Since that time a number of ventilators have been developed in an effort to produce the perfect piece of apparatus.

The main features in maintaining a clear airway, as given by Dr. Lassen, are:

1. High tracheostomy.
2. Well-fitting tracheostomy tube.
3. Humidification.
4. Repeated suction of the trachea and main bronchi.
5. Postural drainage, frequent changes of position and squeezing of the thorax followed by aspiration.

These rules still apply today.

THE ROLE OF THE PHYSIOTHERAPIST

The physiotherapist in the modern intensive care unit, where patients may or may not be receiving artificial ventilation, will be surrounded by a variety of mechanical aids, some of which she will need to use. But her simple basic role is three-fold:

Chest Care

1. To assist in maintaining adequate ventilation by loosening and removing secretions from the lungs.

2. To ensure that the free breathing patient is adequately ventilating all areas of the lungs.

Movement

1. To instruct the patient in free active exercises to maintain mobility and adequate muscle power and aid venous return.

2. To maintain full range joint movement and muscle length by passive movements where the patient is paralysed. This will also aid venous return.

3. To ensure that the positioning of the patient is compatible with the maintenance of good posture.

General Care

1. To have an understanding of the patient, his condition and the medical problems involved.

2. To appreciate the nursing programme and techniques.

THE ROLE OF THE PHYSIOTHERAPIST EXPANDED

The most overwhelming impression when walking into an intensive care unit for the first time is that the room is full of equipment, coupled with a certain amount of mechanical noise. When this is associated with very ill patients and seemingly ultra-efficient staff it can be, for some people, a rather worrying experience. However the equipment is easy to understand, the physiotherapy techniques are basic and there are many people on hand should an emergency arise, which is more than can be said when a cardiac arrest occurs in the street. It is not long before a physiotherapist working on such a unit becomes a skilled member of the team.

The Equipment and its Uses

Standard pieces of equipment, such as ventilators, humidifiers and suction apparatus, have been developed by a number of engineers and doctors. The design will vary in detail but in basic principles of operation each will follow a common pattern. It is only possible to outline these basic principles. Anyone entering an intensive care unit for the first time should familiarize herself with the equipment in that unit and with the routine to be followed in an emergency such as an electrical failure, the breakdown of an individual ventilator, a cardiac arrest or respiratory failure.

ENDOTRACHEAL TUBES, TRACHEOSTOMY TUBES AND AIRWAYS
  (see Fig. 3/1)
The purpose of these tubes is to maintain a clear airway. They were originally made of red rubber, now it is more usual to find that the material used is either Portex (which is a form of plastic) or nylon-reinforced latex.

The *endotracheal tube* is one which passes either through the mouth (oral) or the nose (nasal), the pharynx, the larynx and into the trachea. They vary in size and design. There are two basic oral tubes, the plain and the cuffed, and one, the plain, for use through the nose. The nasal endotracheal tubes are made of much thinner materials than the oral tubes; this allows the lumen to remain as large as for the oral tube but the overall diameter is less. The cuffed oral tube is usually the type chosen, especially for patients on ventilators. When used for artificial ventilation they have a metal connecting piece and in some centres a metal sheath is placed round the outside of the tube between it and the teeth to prevent the patient from biting the tube. Sometimes an airway is placed in the mouth, again to protect the tube. To maintain the endotracheal tube in place a piece of cotton tape is tied firmly round the tube. For easy release this is tied in a bow at the back of the patient's neck.

The use of endotracheal tubes can only be a temporary measure as prolonged intubation may cause inflammation and ulceration of the larynx. It is usually considered that 48 hours is the length of time for safe use but in some cases a period of 72 hours has been tolerated by a patient. However, a tube made of Portex has been used for as long as a week without adverse effect.

There are two types of *tracheostomy tube* in common use, the right-angled cuffed tube made of either Portex or latex and the silver tube. Tracheostomy is an operation, usually performed under a general anaesthetic, in which a short horizontal incision is made in

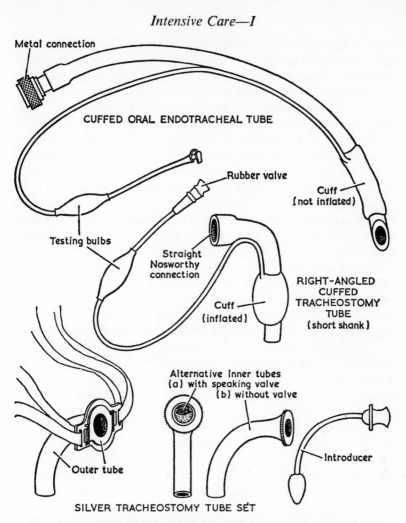

Metal connection

CUFFED ORAL ENDOTRACHEAL TUBE

Rubber valve

Cuff
(not inflated)

Testing bulbs

Straight
Nosworthy
connection

Cuff
(inflated)

RIGHT-ANGLED
CUFFED
TRACHEOSTOMY
TUBE
(short shank)

Alternative inner tubes
(a) with speaking valve
(b) without valve

Outer tube

Introducer

SILVER TRACHEOSTOMY TUBE SET

FIG. 3/1. Diagram showing cuffed endotracheal tube and tracheostomy
tubes (one showing cuff inflated) and standard silver tube

the neck and a small window or fenestra fashioned in the trachea. To
ensure that the tracheostomy tube will be parallel with the walls of
the trachea it is necessary for the surgeon to perform a high tracheostomy at the level of the first and second or second and third tracheal
rings. If the tracheostomy is too low the tube may extend beyond the
carina, enter the right main bronchus and thus prevent air from
entering the left lung. It is normal practice for an endotracheal tube

to be in place during this operation. It is withdrawn to just above the operation site to enable the surgeon to test the tracheostomy tube.

The tracheostomy tube should provide a clear airway with a low resistance to the flow, it should be well-fitting to prevent damage to surrounding structures, and the possibility of accidental displacement should be reduced to a minimum. A right-angled cuffed rubber tube with a metal connecting piece for use with a ventilator was designed by Spalding and Smith in 1956. It is now in common use and called the Radcliffe tracheostomy tube, but present-day materials are used. This tube has a straight arm lying in the trachea, parallel to the walls so that no pressure is exerted on the tissues, and a short section at right angles to this lying in the tracheostome (see Fig. 3/2). The tube is secured in position by a piece of cotton tape fastened round the patient's neck, again in the form of a bow for easy release.

The cuffed form of endotracheal and tracheostomy tube is designed to ensure a good seal between the tube and the trachea. A cuff is a short band of thin latex bonded to the outside of the tube. It can be inflated by a syringe via a small tube which is incorporated into it, one end of which lies outside the patient. Care must be taken not to over-inflate the cuff as pressure on the adjacent structures can cause ulceration by impairing the circulation. Only enough air should be

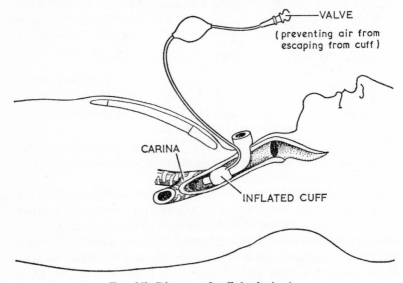

FIG. 3/2. Diagram of cuffed tube in situ

used to create a seal. It is possible, with practice, to judge the correct amount by listening, if necessary with a stethoscope. There should be no audible hissing sound when the patient is receiving artificial ventilation. When the patient is off the ventilator, no air should escape from the mouth or around the tube. A patient with an inflated cuff cannot speak as no air is passing over the vocal cords.

It is necessary to release the air from the cuff from time to time to remove the pressure on the trachea and to clear secretions which have collected round the tube. The frequency with which this is done varies from centre to centre; in some instances it is released four-hourly. Others feel that regular release of the cuff is unnecessary and it is only done when the tube is changed or to allow the patient to speak. If the patient cannot swallow, this procedure should be carried out with his head down below the horizontal.

The release of the cuff is of particular importance to the paralysed patient to allow him to speak and make his needs known. However expert one is at lip-reading one cannot always understand what a patient is saying. The patient who is not paralysed will be able to communicate by writing.

Some right-angled tracheostomy tubes are designed with a long cuff and this ensures a larger area of contact and reduces the possibility of undue pressure being exerted at any point. Another tube has been produced which has two cuffs which can be inflated alternately.

The functions of the cuffed tube are:

1. To prevent substances from the mouth from entering the lungs.

2. To help to maintain positive pressure ventilation by preventing air from escaping round the tube.

3. To reduce the dead air space, thus facilitating ventilation of the lungs by the free breathing patient.

There is a standard set of sizes for the Radcliffe Tracheostomy Tubes numbered Magill sizes 4, 6, 8, 10 and 12. These are available in two types called the long and short shank.

The usual metal connections between the endotracheal tube or a tracheostomy tube and the ventilator are called Nosworthy connections, straight and curved. To prevent them from separating accidentally, in some centres they are magnetised and in others a small screw is incorporated which can be released when it is necessary to disconnect the patient.

The silver tracheostomy tube cannot be used for connection to a ventilator and is used in the intermediate stage before finally closing the tracheostomy. It is sometimes a permanent feature for patients following laryngectomy. It usually has an inner tube which can be removed for cleaning. Some have a valve which allows the patient with a larynx to speak.

The disadvantages of tracheostomy are the increased danger of infection and the loss of humidification. Dry gases entering the trachea can cause crusts to form and a blockage of one of the respiratory passages may occur.

Both endotracheal and tracheostomy tubes facilitate the aspiration of secretions from the trachea.

Opinions differ as to the frequency with which tracheostomy tubes should be changed. Within a few days of operation there is a firm track from the skin to the trachea and after this there is usually no difficulty in changing the tube.

Occasionally it may be necessary to use an *airway* to facilitate suction through the mouth. All physiotherapists should be familiar with the airway, which is frequently in position when a patient returns from theatre. It is a simple tube, usually made of rigid plastic, flattened vertically, with a metal flange to prevent it from slipping past the teeth and into the mouth completely. It has a right-angled bend, so that the tube fits over the tongue and down into the pharynx. Airways vary in size. An airway cannot be used for artificial ventilation. It serves the simple purpose of preventing the tongue from falling backwards and suffocating the unconscious patient; it also gives a clear pathway for suction in both the conscious and the unconscious patient. In some centres individual physiotherapists after tuition are allowed to insert them without supervision. The usual method of doing this is to put the airway into the mouth with the curved end pointing upwards. Once in the mouth it is rotated through 180°. It is then in position to restrain the tongue, protect the suction catheter from being bitten and direct it into the pharynx.

HUMIDIFICATION

Humidification is the moistening of the air or gases we breathe. This is one of the functions of the upper part of the respiratory tract.

Artificial humidification is necessary for patients in the following circumstances:

1. When breathing through endotracheal or tracheostomy tubes. The natural humidification and warming function of the upper respiratory tract is bypassed if a patient is breathing either through an endotracheal or tracheostomy tube. Dry air at lower than body temperature passing over secretions in the bronchial tree extracts moisture from them causing crusts to be formed. These crusts may partially block the trachea or main bronchus or occlude one of the smaller airways. They are very difficult to remove. Artificial humidification is essential for the maintenance of adequate ventilation in this situation.

The vast majority of ventilators incorporate some form of humidification. Patients who have a permanent silver tracheostomy tube seem to acclimatize themselves to the lack of humidification and provided the inner tube is cleaned regularly suffer no gross ill-effects.

2. When breathing air to which gases have been added.

These gases are completely dry and will require considerable humidification and it may be considered advantageous to the patient to augment the natural humidification process.

3. When secretions are abnormally thick. Humidification will facilitate their removal.

There are several methods of achieving humidification, but the majority have the same two problems to a greater or lesser extent.

Condensation in the tubes is one of these and when using apparatus where this pertains, care must be taken to ensure that the tubes are emptied at regular intervals. It is very distressing for the patient when water enters a tracheostomy tube. The other problem is that humidifiers are liable to become infected by bacteria and introduce this infection into the patient's respiratory system. Careful sterilisation of apparatus is essential.

METHODS OF HUMIDIFICATION

1. Bernoulli Effect. In this method a jet of air is blown across a fine tube set in a bath of water. Water in the form of both vapour and droplets is drawn up the tube and carried away as a fine mist. Although the larger particles are removed before the air reaches the delivery tube there is considerable condensation especially in the heated models.

2. Condenser. In this method no water is added to the gases which reach the patient but the vapour which is contained in the expired air is condensed out on a wire mesh, usually made of gold, silver or cupro-nickle. On the next inspiration some of this condensed water is picked up as droplets. This method is aimed at preventing the loss of moisture and is probably only of use as a temporary measure. It is frequently used in theatre.

3. Water-Bath Humidifiers.

a) Bubble-through. As the name suggests air or gases are bubbled through a water bath collecting moisture on the way. An example of this is the Wolfe bottle. Some authorities do not consider this method to be very effective.

b) Steam kettle. This type of humidifier usually incorporates a fan which blows air across the surface of a water bath containing a heating element, the temperature of which can be regulated and the water maintained at between 37–60° C. The air or gases which leave the humidifier are fully saturated at the set temperature.

The main problem with this type is that considerable condensation occurs and that, although the temperature of the humidified air leaving the kettle is known, the temperature after it has passed through the delivery tube is difficult to control. The best temperature to be achieved is 33° C in the trachea.

The hot water has the effect of killing bacteria. All the humidification produced with the steam kettle method is in the form of a vapour which is not effective in loosening thick secretions. Droplets are required for this. The East Radcliffe is an example of the steam kettle type of humidifier (see Fig. 3/3 (a)).

4. Ultrasonic Nebulizers (see Fig. 3/3 (b)). Humidification is produced in a nebulizer by water dropping on to a high speed rotating metal plate or vibrating crystal. One drop at a time the water is shattered into micro-droplets. These droplets can be extremely small and 97% may be up to 1–5 microns in diameter (Chaney, 1969).

Because large quantities of droplets are produced, this form of humidification is very effective in loosening sticky secretions.

The disadvantages with this method are:

a) Nebulizers easily become infected and because of the minute droplets produced, infection is taken far into the respiratory system.

b) It is difficult to maintain a constant drip.

c) There is no way of completely regulating the degree of humidity and over-humidification could be dangerous. In effect a patient could drown.

5. In some centres during chest clearance when the secretions are very thick and difficult to remove, the physiotherapist will

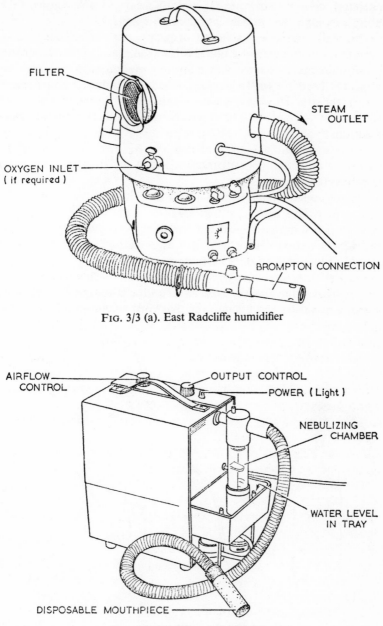

FILTER

STEAM OUTLET

OXYGEN INLET
(if required)

BROMPTON CONNECTION

Fig. 3/3 (a). East Radcliffe humidifier

AIRFLOW CONTROL

OUTPUT CONTROL

POWER (Light)

NEBULIZING CHAMBER

WATER LEVEL IN TRAY

DISPOSABLE MOUTHPIECE

Fig. 3/3 (b). Ultrasonic nebulizer

introduce *normal saline* into the endotracheal or tracheostomy tube using a syringe. The maximum quantity is 2 ml.

Distilled water and a solution of bicarbonate of soda have also been used for this purpose but it is believed that distilled water can cause pulmonary oedema and a strong solution of bicarbonate of soda has been shown to damage mucous membrane and depress ciliary activity. However, a very weak solution of bicarbonate of soda at pH 7·4 may be safe to use. Normal saline is a physiological solution.

METHODS BY WHICH HUMIDIFIED AIR CAN BE INTRODUCED INTO THE RESPIRATORY SYSTEM

    1. A free breathing patient who is not intubated.

      a) A face mask (see Fig. 3/4).

      b) A mouthpiece which the patient has to hold. This method is frequently used with a nebulizer as a method of giving a short period of humidification prior to chest clearance.

    2. A free breathing patient with a tracheostomy tube (see Fig. 3/5).

      a) A tracheostomy humidifying tube (Brompton tube). This is made of plastic and fits into the Nosworthy connection.

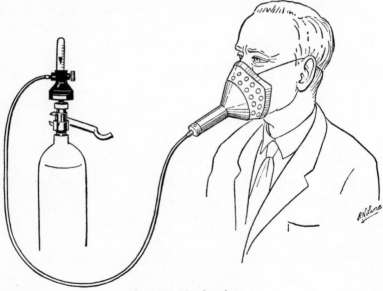

FIG. 3/4. Ventimask

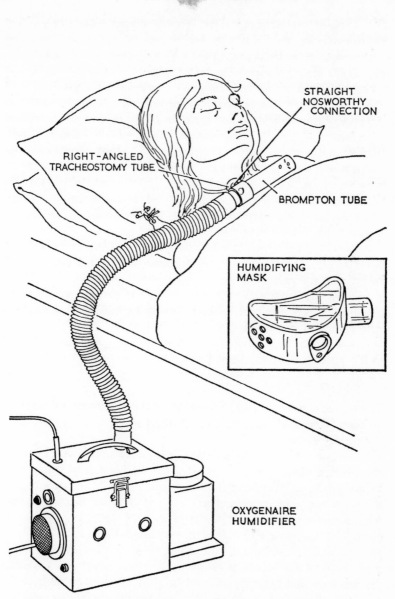

FIG. 3/5. Tracheostomy tube in situ and Oxygenaire humidifier. Inset is
shown a humidifying mask

b) A tracheostomy mask. This is a rigid plastic box which fits over the tracheostomy tube and is secured by a tape either tied round the neck or fixed to the pillow by a piece of tape and a safety-pin. There are also disposable flexible plastic covers.

3. A patient on intermittent positive pressure ventilation.

A humidifier is usually incorporated into the ventilator.

Types of humidification and methods of use will vary from centre to centre but there are two points which should be considered. Firstly, should the humidified air be heated? Many people consider that it is necessary to have the humidified air heated to a temperature between 30–36° C for patients whose upper respiratory tract has been bypassed. Secondly, what type of humidification is most advantageous for a particular patient, vapour or droplets? Vapour is ineffective in loosening thick sticky secretions.

Because it is not possible to completely regulate the degree of humidification in the ultrasonic nebulizer care must be taken to ensure that the patient is not over-humidified. A method of control is to limit the duration and frequency of the periods spent on the nebulizer; this is particularly applicable to the free breathing patient with copious sticky sputum.

Drugs such as bronchodilators and mucolytic agents may be added to the water in the nebulizers.

SUCTION

The frequent removal of secretions from the respiratory passages is an essential part of the treatment of the patient requiring intensive respiratory care.

Some patients will be able to cough at either a voluntary or reflex level, others will not. It is unusual for the very ill patient who is able to cough and co-operate in the treatment, to be able to do so effectively enough to maintain a clear airway at all times. Secretions may remain in the pharynx. Suction will then be necessary to remove them. If it is necessary to induce the patient to cough at a reflex level suction will again be required to remove the secretions. Other patients, who are unable to cough either because they are so deeply unconscious that the reflex cannot be stimulated or because of the paralysis of the expiratory muscles, will require suction to clear the secretions which have been moved from the lungs by postural drainage and manual techniques.

Suction should be given:

1. Whenever secretions can be heard.
2. Before and after a change of position.
3. Before and during the release of the cuff.
4. If the patient looks distressed and changes colour.
5. If the minute volume drops. (*Minute volume* is the amount of air either inspired or expired in one minute. It is usual to measure the M.V. of expired air as this is considered to be a more reliable guide.) It is usually taken and recorded hourly by the nursing staff using a volume meter. The level of the M.V. should be noted by the physiotherapist before and after the treatment as it is an indication as to the state of the patient.

SUCTION APPARATUS

Suction Pumps (see Fig. 3/6)

Nature abhors a vacuum and does its best to fill it. This is the principle upon which suction apparatus is built. There are four basic types of apparatus which may be classified according to the power used to create the vacuum or suction force. This vacuum is filled simultaneously with its production, by substances (air, water, sputum, blood) passing down the suction tube.

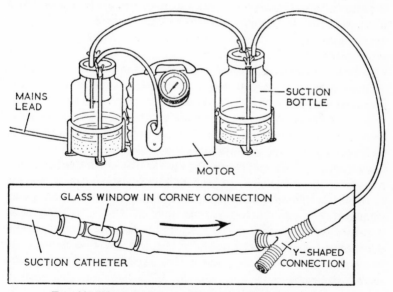

MAINS LEAD

SUCTION BOTTLE

MOTOR

GLASS WINDOW IN CORNEY CONNECTION

SUCTION CATHETER

Y–SHAPED CONNECTION

FIG. 3/6. Diagram of suction apparatus. Inset are Y-shaped and Corney connections with suction catheter attached

1. Electrical suction apparatus which is powered from the mains. This type has its own small motor with an on/off switch.

2. Suction apparatus designed to work from a vacuum point adjacent to the patient's bed; again there is an on/off switch. The power in this instance is provided by a large motor situated at some convenient site within the hospital grounds.

3. Foot pump: here as the name suggests, the power is provided by the individual operator. This type of pump was the only one available in the period when intensive care was developing. Today a foot pump is rarely used but one should be available in case of a power failure.

4. Occasionally one may find suction apparatus working from a gas cylinder. Again this is usually a piece of emergency equipment.

Each suction pump has either one or two suction bottles, depending upon the design, partially filled with some antiseptic solution. The connecting tubes enter through the lid which is secured in such a way as to prevent leakage. Usually the lid is maintained in position by two metal clamps controlled by screws (see Fig. 3/6).

The suction tube leads from a bottle to the stem of a Y-shaped semi-transparent plastic connection, the purpose of which is to control the suction. One arm is open and onto the other is attached a short piece of tubing which leads to a connection for attachment of the suction catheter. It is an advantage if this second connection is made partly of glass. The Corney connection is frequently used (see Fig. 3/6). It takes the form of a glass cylinder enclosed in a metal framework with a tapered end to which the catheter is attached. The operator can then take note of the type of secretions passing through the tube. A connection made entirely of glass would break too easily. In some centres the suction catheter is attached directly to the Y-shaped connection: this has two disadvantages. Firstly it is difficult to attach the catheter to the plastic arm which frequently has a relatively large diameter, and secondly the plastic is rather opaque. A rigid transparent plastic suction end made in the form of an elongated tube with a hole at the proximal end to control the suction is now being introduced. It will serve a dual purpose as its elongated shape makes it suitable for mouth suction and a suction catheter can be fixed to the end. This may in time replace the Y-shaped and Corney connections.

If the apparatus has not been used for some time or if it has only just been cleaned, it is advisable to test it with water before use. If suction is not adequate it is wise to check the lids of the bottles to see that they are well screwed down and to inspect all the tube connections. It is even possible that the on/off switch could be in the wrong position.

Catheters

Whistle-tipped soft rubber catheters sizes 9–12 French gauge are used. To minimize the damage to the mucous membrane it is essential that the catheters should be made of a soft flexible material; rubber is commonly used but a soft plastic disposable catheter is now being developed. The catheter must have two holes close together on opposite sides of the suction end. If one hole becomes adherent to the mucous membrane of the respiratory tract, the resistance at that point will be greater than at the unobstructed hole. Therefore, air will pass through this hole and the suction force exerted on the membrane will be contained.

Bronchoscopy or Pinkerton's catheters should be available on the unit for selective suction of the left main bronchus which is occasionally necessary. Normally if a soft rubber suction catheter descends beyond the carina it will enter the right main bronchus which is almost a direct continuation of the trachea. If the head is side flexed to the right there is a greater chance of the catheter entering the left main bronchus. If the left main bronchus is blocked by secretions, it is necessary to use a Pinkerton's catheter which has a curved end of hardened rubber. In skilled hands this can be directed into the left main bronchus, a mark on the other end of the catheter indicating the position of the curve.

In common with much other equipment, catheters arrive on the ward in packs from the Central Sterilising Supply Unit (C.S.S.U.). There should be an unlimited supply of these. The number in a pack will vary but when opened the contents should be emptied into a sterile bowl with the help of forceps. In some units it is still necessary for the ward to sterilise its own catheters by boiling. Before sterilising in this manner the catheters should be washed and tied into one bundle for easy handling. Usually at least 24 will be required for each patient. All catheters must only be used once and then placed with the other unsterile catheters in a separate bowl.

Suction Trolley (see Fig. 3/7)

The layout of the suction trolley will vary in detail but it should have:

1. Packet of disposable gloves.
2. Forceps in a container filled with antiseptic fluid.
3. Bowl for gauze swabs.
4. Tube of lubricating jelly.
5. Two or three bowls with lids, one containing sterile catheters, another containing a solution of bicarbonate of soda, which is passed through the catheter after suction to clear the sputum and act as a solvent, and a third containing antiseptic solution into which the catheters are discarded. In some instances the catheters will be discarded into the bowl containing the bicarbonate of soda solution.

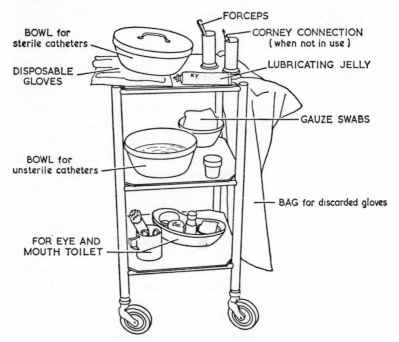

FIG. 3/7. Diagram of suction trolley

6. A metal container filled with antiseptic solution in which the Corney connection may be placed after use and a bulldog clip to fix the suction tube onto the rail of the trolley. Sometimes the connection is kept inside a sterile plastic glove.
7. Plastic bag fixed with adhesive tape onto the trolley for discarded gloves.

8. Suction apparatus (this may be fixed to the wall).

9. In some centres the operator wears a face mask. In that case there will be a box of masks on the trolley.

Preparing to aspirate. On all occasions a 'no touch' technique must be adopted as the risk of introducing infection into the respiratory tract is high. Methods of doing this will vary from unit to unit and the physiotherapist should adopt the method advocated by the medical personnel in charge of the unit in which she is working.

In one unit the procedure is as follows:

1. Wash the hands before starting the treatment and if necessary before preparing to aspirate.

2. Switch on the suction apparatus. It is never easy to do this later unless the on/off switch is foot operated.

3. Squeeze a quantity of sterile lubricating jelly onto a sterile swab. Catheters boiled on the ward are kept in sterile water which keeps them well lubricated but catheters from the C.S.S.U. packs are dry. Sterilised glycerin was used as a method of lubrication but it was found to be an irritant.

4. Put a glove either onto the dominant hand (right) or usually on both.

5. Release the bulldog clip with the left hand and remove the Corney connection from its container with the right.

6. Transfer the suction tube to the left hand and hold it at the Y-shaped connection.

7. Remove the lid of the bowl containing sterile catheters with the left hand which continues to hold the Y-shaped connection. This will be achieved with a little practice.

8. Using forceps in the right hand select a sterile catheter and lift the end to be attached to the connection from the bowl. It is advisable to leave the suction tip in the bowl.

9. Still using the forceps attach the catheter to the Corney connection.

10. Remove the catheter from the bowl with the forceps, holding it a little above the suction tip. If the catheter is to be introduced via the nose or mouth it is necessary to hold it in the gloved hand.

11. Replace the lid of the bowl.

12. Finally pass the suction tip of the catheter through the sterile jelly or sterile water.

Ways of entry for a suction catheter. There are three possible routes by which a suction catheter may be introduced into the respiratory tract: the nose, the mouth and via a tube. Passing a catheter, particularly via the nose and mouth is a very uncomfortable procedure for the conscious patient. It must be done with the correct combination of gentleness and firmness. This is the direct product of the attitude of mind of the operator. Fear or distaste for the job in hand will result in either ineffective or over-vigorous use of the catheter. If possible, it is advisable to make one's first attempts at suction in this way on an unconscious patient. He will not be distressed and the operator can gain that confidence which is necessary to use any form of apparatus efficiently.

1. When using the nose as a mode of entry the patient's neck is extended so that the head is tilted backwards resting on a pillow. A lubricated catheter is held between the fingers and thumb of a gloved hand and introduced into the nose. It is directed slightly upwards and backwards until the tip reaches the posterior naris where a little resistance may be felt. A way through can usually be found by carefully rolling the catheter between the index finger and thumb. If the patient has a Ryle's tube in position it has been found in practice easier to use the same nostril. The catheter seems to slide along the first tube and through the posterior naris easily.

The catheter then enters the pharynx. The position of the catheter beyond this point cannot be determined accurately. It may curl up in the mouth but this is a rare occurrence and it can be seen. Some authorities doubt if the catheter reaches beyond the pharynx and into the upper part of the bronchial tree but the fact remains that on some occasions a cough reflex can be elicited and on others the patient begins to retch. It is certain that if the patient is conscious and able to co-operate by taking deep breaths with the mouth open and the catheter is only advanced during inspiration, a cough reflex can be stimulated in the majority of cases. By using this method of advancing the catheter during inspiration even in the unconscious patient success is achieved in a high percentage of attempts.

The nose is a very successful way of entering a suction catheter into the respiratory tract. Unfortunately for the patients it is very uncomfortable but if they are well prepared and able to co-operate the majority tolerate it extremely well.

2. The mouth is a relatively unsatisfactory mode of entry unless the patient is extremely co-operative and even then it may be necessary to use a lubricated airway. The mouth is such a large cavity that it is easy to misdirect the catheter and it is not unusual to see the

suction end appear again between the teeth. The patient may bite the catheter unless an airway is used.

3. The introduction of a catheter into either an endotracheal or a tracheostomy tube using a pair of forceps presents no difficulties. However, it must be remembered that if a patient is dependent upon a ventilator the time available for suction is strictly limited. To get some idea of a patient's tolerance one should exhale as far as possible and note how long one can remain comfortable without taking a breath.

Suction. Unless the patient is very restless catheters are always introduced into an endotracheal or a tracheostomy tube using a pair of forceps.

The catheter is advanced as far as possible, care being taken to ensure that suction does not take place during the entry phase. Considerable damage has been shown to be done to the mucous membrane even by the most skilful operator and suction on the way in is considered to be especially traumatic. The Y-shaped connection is designed to prevent this. The open arm of the Y offers less resistance to the suction force than does the catheter. The suction apparatus therefore takes the line of least resistance and air is taken in through the open arm. If the Y-shaped connection is not available the catheter itself can be pinched to prevent suction from taking place.

Having advanced the catheter as far as possible the forceps are returned to their container and the catheter held between the finger and thumb of the gloved hand. Suction is started by occluding the open arm of the Y-shaped connection with the thumb of the other hand. The catheter is then slowly and gently withdrawn using intermittent suction. As it is removed it is rotated first one way and then the other between the finger and thumb. If a pool of secretions is reached, there is a pause until it is clear, always remembering the time factor for the patient dependent upon a ventilator. Under no circumstances should the 'tromboning' method be used, *i.e.* a vigorous up and down movement.

If the catheter appears to be blocked it is occasionally possible to clear it by moving the thumb off and on the open arm of the Y-shaped connection.

After suction the ventilator patient is re-attached immediately.

The suction end of the catheter is then placed into the bowl containing a solution of bicarbonate of soda and cleared. It is then discarded and the connection returned to its holder, the suction tube secured, the bowls re-covered and the glove removed.

If a specimen of sputum is required for bacteriological study a special sputum trap can be fitted in between the Corney connection and the suction catheter.

INTERMITTENT POSITIVE PRESSURE VENTILATION (I.P.P.V.)
In patients who are receiving I.P.P.V., inspiration occurs when air under positive pressure (above atmospheric pressure) enters the lungs. Air continues to flow until the pressure in the airway is equal to the elastic resistance of the lungs and the weight of the chest wall. As the intrathoracic pressure is raised above atmospheric pressure the pressure gradient between the periphery and the right atrium hinders venous return. It is possible to switch a negative pressure

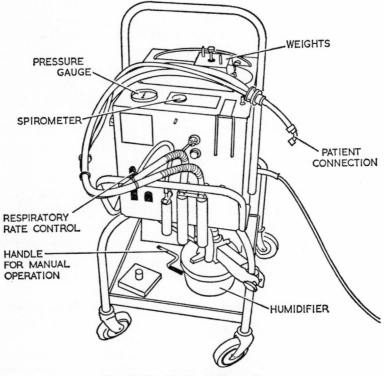

FIG. 3/8 (a). The Radcliffe ventilator

phase into the expiratory cycle of the majority of ventilators to assist the circulation, if this is deemed advisable by the medical staff.

Following the development of the original method of I.P.P.V. many machines have been produced. It is usual to classify them as time cycled, volume cycled and pressure cycled. This classification refers to the inspiratory phase.

In a *time-cycled* ventilator the rate and duration of inspiration and expiration are pre-set. The Radcliffe (see Fig. 3/8 (a)) and the Barnet are examples of this type. The volume of air or gases delivered to the patient depends upon the force with which they are driven in. In the Radcliffe this pressure is provided by variable weights on top of a bellows which utilizes room air: oxygen can be fed into the ventilator. The Barnet uses gases either piped from a central supply or from cylinders. Some Barnet ventilators can be triggered by the patient on demand. The time-cycled ventilator is usually the method chosen for longterm cases. The Radcliffe runs off mains electricity and has a car-type accumulator for use during a power failure or when transporting the patient. It can also be operated by hand. The Barnet requires electricity to control the circuit and to charge the battery continuously. The battery will last 24 hours when fully charged.

A *volume-cycled* ventilator is one in which inspiration ends when a

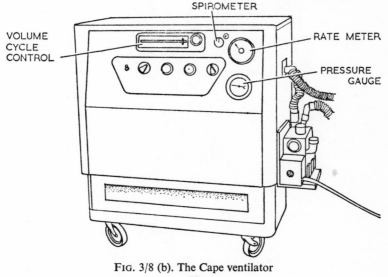

Fig. 3/8 (b). The Cape ventilator

pre-set volume has been delivered. An example of this is the Cape
ventilator (see Fig. 3/8 (b)). Pressure readings can be made during
the inflation period and reflect both the lung compliance and the
resistance of the delivery tubing. They are only indirectly related to
the volumes of gases actually delivered to the patient. Either a block
in the tubes or changes in the lung compliance will be shown by
alterations in the reading. The machine can be operated by hand.

Examples of *pressure-cycled* ventilators are the Bennett and the
Bird. This type of ventilator operates to a pre-determined pressure
and when this pressure of gas is reached in the patient's lungs and
the tubes leading to him, the flow of gas is cut off and expiration
occurs. Of these the Bird is probably the most popular (see Fig. 3/8
(c) and (d)). The Bird Mark 7 or 8 is powered by gas under pressure.

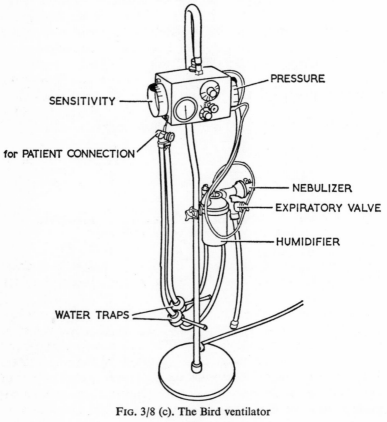

Fig. 3/8 (c). The Bird ventilator

It can be connected either to a cylinder or to a piped system of oxygen or compressed air. When air is used as the driving force oxygen may be added, or if oxygen is used as the driving force 100% oxygen or a mixture of oxygen and entrained atmospheric air can be given. This mixture is reputedly 40% oxygen though it may prove to be considerably higher. The ventilator can be cycled automatically or be set to be triggered by the free-breathing patient who requires assistance. The sensitivity control can be finely adjusted so that the slightest inspiratory effort by the patient producing a small negative pressure within the ventilator will trigger the inspiratory phase. If required the ventilator can be operated manually.

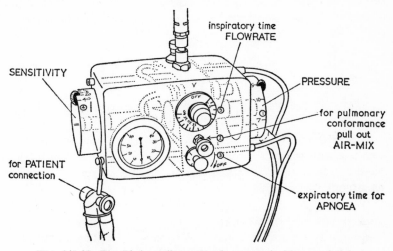

FIG. 3/8 (d). The Bird ventilator showing controls. Names of dials are of course printed on the instrument

Oxygen can be fed into all ventilators and a humidifier is either built into the original design or it can be incorporated into the circuit.

The physiotherapist will not be required to adjust the ventilator and set the controls. This is usually done by the anaesthetist or physician in charge but she should be able to identify the controls and read the dials, although the records will be kept by the nursing staff. The only exception to this is when the Bird is being used as part of the chest clearance programme (see Chapter 5 on intermittent positive pressure breathing). However she should know how to transfer a ventilator from mains to battery power or how to operate it manually should the occasion arise.

The patient with an endotracheal or tracheostomy tube will be connected to the ventilator by tubes with Nosworthy straight and curved connections (see Fig. 3/8 (e)). These connecting tubes can be quite heavy and if not carefully adjusted can pull most uncomfortably on the tracheostomy tube. In some centres an adjustable arm, clamped to the bed frame at the head of the patient, is used to take the strain. The tubes are attached to it by cotton tape. Another method, which is not quite as effective, is to attach the tubes to the sheet or pillow, if used, by cotton tape and a safety-pin or artery forceps.

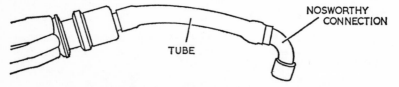

FIG. 3/8 (e). The curved Nosworthy connection

The Bird ventilator is not always used in conjunction with an endotracheal or tracheostomy tube. It can be used with a mouthpiece or a face mask (see Chapter 5 on intermittent positive pressure breathing).

ADMINISTRATION OF OXYGEN

The majority of patients in an intensive care unit will require oxygen-enriched air. The amount required will be assessed by the anaesthetist or physician and his judgement will be made firstly by the clinical appearance of the patient and secondly by laboratory analysis of a blood sample which will give the pCO_2, pO_2 and the pH.

Patients receiving I.P.P.V. will receive oxygen through the ventilator. Free-breathing patients with endotracheal or tracheostomy tubes will receive humidified oxygen and air either through a box type tracheostomy mask or through a tracheostomy humidifying tube (see Fig. 3/5, page 67). With this tube the patient can receive approximately 100% oxygen with the hole opposite to the tracheostomy tube closed or approximately 50% oxygen with the hole open.

Oxygen is administered to patients without a tracheostomy or endotracheal tube via a face mask (see Fig. 3/4, page 66) or nasal spectacles. There is quite a selection of masks available but the following table will list the more common ones and the approximate percentage of oxygen delivered to the patient. Concentrations are variable depending on the oxygen flow. Instructions come with the masks.

% of Oxygen	Apparatus	O_2 Flow Rate per minute
100%	anaesthetic mask	
80%	B.L.B. mask	6–8 litres
60–70%	Edinburgh mask + snout	6 litres
50%	Edinburgh mask	4 litres
24% & 28%	Ventimask	4 litres
35%	Ventimask	8 litres
?	Nasal spectacles	2–4 litres

The amount of oxygen received by a patient wearing nasal spectacles is difficult to assess as he is not obliged to breathe consistently through the nose. He is free to breathe through the mouth, in which case he will not be receiving oxygen-enriched air. They are nevertheless the device best tolerated by patients.

It is always a temptation to increase the oxygen being given to a patient who is distressed and looks very hypoxic. However, it must always be remembered that the administration of excessive quantities of oxygen can have a depressing effect on respiration especially in patients with chronic diffuse airways obstruction.

ANALGESIA

The use of analgesia to facilitate chest clearance is of particular value in the post-operative care of patients who have had a thoracotomy. These patients are conscious, co-operative and able to cough voluntarily. Coughing is a very tiring and painful process and on occasions it may be necessary to assist a patient by administering a mild analgesic. The physiotherapist must have been authorized to do this. The type of patient particularly helped is one who has a chronic bronchitis or asthma prior to surgery. He is required to do more than the normal amount of coughing post-operatively.

There are two types of analgesia commonly available and both are used with a face mask in which there is a patient-triggered demand valve. Care must be taken to ensure that, when holding the mask to the face, the patient achieves a good seal and that he inspires deeply enough to trigger the valve. This can be heard in action.

With the Entonox apparatus, the patient is breathing a mixture of 50% nitrous oxide and 50% oxygen which is contained in a cylinder fixed onto a trolley for easy transportation. The patient is asked to breathe deeply for up to one minute or to take 10 to 12 deep breaths. The mask is then removed and the patient assisted to cough. The analgesic effect lasts up to five minutes.

The Cardiff inhaler in which Penthrane is used is small enough to go into a box about 2 ft by 1 ft which will also hold the bottle of liquid Penthrane and the tube for filling the inhaler. The patient is asked to breathe deeply using the mask for five minutes. He will then be relatively pain-free for up to twenty minutes.

There seem to be no side-effects with either Entonox or Penthrane although Penthrane has been known to cause kidney disease following anaesthesia.

Care must be taken to prevent cross-infection either by having several masks or by cleaning the mask after use.

It is essential that the patient should fully understand what is being done and why; some people are very afraid of having a mask over the face.

Unfortunately a small proportion of patients do not find this an effective method of relieving pain.

RECORDS AND PATIENT MONITORING

The purpose of the intensive care unit is to ensure that the patient receives the best care, treatment and supervision. Records must be kept so that a clear picture of the patient's condition can easily be appreciated by all the staff.

Methods and charts will vary from unit to unit but it is usual to record the following: minute volume, respiratory rate, pressure readings from the ventilator, size of tracheostomy tube, blood pressure, pulse, temperature and level of consciousness of the patient. Space will also be allocated on which drugs and treatments including physiotherapy and times of X-ray, etc. may be recorded. A fluid chart may be necessary and the diet indicated.

Regular blood samples will be taken for testing by the laboratory staff. It is necessary to know if the patient is being adequately ventilated and this is reflected in the oxygen and carbon dioxide tension in the arterial blood. The process of blood gas analysis and the assessment of the acid-base balance used to be a long and complicated process. A much speedier method has been developed by Dr. P.

Astrup, a Danish biochemist, and his colleagues. The apparatus, the Micro Astrup apparatus, which is named after its inventor, can produce the necessary information from a small sample of capillary or arterial blood.

The television type of monitor, giving a continuous E.C.G. tracing, will be found in the Cardiac Surgery, Coronary Care and Respiratory Care Units.

X-rays, which in many cases will be taken routinely, may be displayed on a viewing box and should be studied prior to treatment.

EMERGENCY PROCEDURES

i) Failure of Power Supply

As already indicated it is necessary for all the staff of an intensive care unit to be familiar with the means by which the ventilators in that unit, using electrical power, can be changed from mains to battery or operated by hand. In case the power failure occurs in the hours of darkness there should be emergency lighting available. Some hospitals have an alternative power supply.

ii) Respiratory Arrest

Following respiratory arrest the first-aid treatment is mouth-to-mouth breathing.

The basis for the effectiveness of this method is that the gases of the dead air space do not reach the level of gaseous exchange. Inspired air contains 21% oxygen and no carbon dioxide, alveolar air contains 14% oxygen and 6% carbon dioxide, and expired air, which is a mixture of alveolar air and the inspired air of the dead space, contains 16% oxygen and 4% carbon dioxide. This expired air contains enough oxygen to maintain an adequate level of oxygenation and the carbon dioxide level remains low enough to be unimportant so that it is possible to keep the patient alive for a considerable time.

Method

1. Place the patient in a supine lying position if convenient but mouth-to-mouth breathing should be started as soon as possible, *e.g.* while he is being carried out of the sea or river.

2. Make sure that the mouth is clear of substances which may obstruct the airway, for example, vomit or seaweed. The head should be extended and the jaw pulled forwards by placing the fingers behind the angle of the jaw, so that the tongue is brought forwards and prevented from falling backwards and obstructing the airway.

3. Working from the side, place the mouth over the patient's mouth and ensure that leakage does not occur. It is necessary to close off the patient's nose. This may be done by the cheek but it is more effective to pinch the nose between the fingers and thumb of the hand not supporting the jaw. In a small child the mouth is placed over both the mouth and nose of the patient.

Some people prefer mouth-to-nose breathing and this may be the only possible method if the jaw muscles are in spasm.

4. The operator then blows gently into the patient's mouth until the ribs rise. N.B. This should not be a hard blow. To allow the patient to expire and the operator to inspire the mouth is removed from the patient's face.

5. Rate 10–20 times/minute.

6. Mouth-to-mouth breathing should continue until the patient is breathing adequately or until a more competent person makes the decision that further attempts at resuscitation should stop.

The importance of speed in starting operations cannot be over-stressed.

If all other methods of ventilating a patient who is dependent upon mechanical aid fails, the staff should be prepared to do mouth-to-tracheostomy breathing. In fact mouth-to-tracheostomy breathing which follows the same pattern as mouth-to-mouth breathing is easier, as, with the cuff inflated air will not escape. It cannot be said that this is a pleasant or desirable process because the patient is likely to have a chest infection. The unit should be equipped with a supply of Ambu Resuscitators or self-inflating bags (see Fig. 3/9).

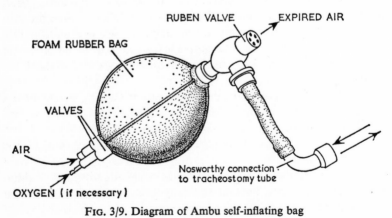

RUBEN VALVE   EXPIRED AIR

FOAM RUBBER BAG

VALVES

AIR

Nosworthy connection to tracheostomy tube

OXYGEN (if necessary)

Fig. 3/9. Diagram of Ambu self-inflating bag

The Ambu Resuscitator is basically a rubber bag with foam rubber walls. The foam rubber causes the bag to return to its original shape and size after manual compression. Air enters through a non-return valve and expired air passes through a Ruben valve which avoids re-breathing. The Ambu can be connected to a tracheostomy tube by a short piece of corrugated rubber tubing and a Nosworthy connection.

On the same principle of avoiding actual patient contact, if possible, when there is the likelihood of chest infection, a Brook Airway with a one-way valve should be used in hospital for mouth-to-mouth breathing.

iii) Cardiac Arrest
Signs of cardiac arrest.
    a) Absence of palpable carotid pulses.
    b) Pallor or cyanosis of the skin—a sudden deterioration.
    c) Rapidly dilating pupils—a sign of cerebral hypoxia.

When applying external cardiac massage one is intermittently compressing the heart between the sternum and the thoracic vertebrae. When compression is given, blood is expelled from the heart into the pulmonary arteries and the aorta; when pressure is released the blood in the main veins enters the heart.

Method

1. Place the patient in a supine position on a hard surface. All beds in an intensive care unit should be of the solid base design or have fracture boards. Failing this the patient should be put onto the floor.

2. The operator stands or kneels by the patient so that he can apply pressure through straight arms.

3. The heel of one hand is put over the heel of the other and both are placed over the sternum. Accuracy at this moment is very important. The point for compression is identified by palpating the xiphisternal end of the body of the sternum and pressure is given a little above the point at which the sternum can be felt to spring back, *i.e.* the upper part of the lower half of the sternum. Another method of identifying the point for compression is to measure one index finger length down from the sternal angle, allowing a little more for small hands.

4. The weight should be applied vertically through straight arms. With children it may be necessary to use the fingers or the heel of one hand.

Too much pressure, especially in an incorrect position, can lead to fractured ribs; too little is ineffective. If a second person is available he should palpate the carotid pulses.

5. Rate—approximately 80 per minute.

iv) Resuscitation

If the operator is working alone and the patient is not breathing, the first act is to clear the airway.

The proportion of mouth-to-mouth breathing and external cardiac massage is one breath to 6 to 8 compressions of the chest.

It is more satisfactory to have two people working together, in which case care must be taken to ensure that compression does not occur at the same time as the patient is being given a breath.

In the hospital situation help will always be quickly available; on an intensive care unit it will be immediately to hand.

If the physiotherapist in this first-aid situation should start resuscitation she should continue until more experienced staff bringing drugs and defibrillating equipment reach the patient.

In most hospitals a plastic model will be available to enable the staff to practise these techniques. This practice is very useful and gives a certain amount of confidence.

For references and bibliography, see end of Chapter 4.

CHAPTER 4

Intensive Care—II

by P. J. WADDINGTON, M.C.S.P., H.T., DIP.T.P.

TECHNIQUES OF CHEST CLEARANCE

Positioning

The positioning of a patient so that gravity contributes to chest clearance is a standard procedure. A knowledge of the basic postural drainage positions (see page 114) is essential to any physiotherapist doing chest work. However, in the intensive care unit to be able to position the patient accurately for all the bronchopulmonary segments is the exception rather than the rule, for either the patient's condition or the mere fact that he is on a ventilator will prevent it.

The patient with a head injury may or may not be put into a head down position because of the possibility of raising intracranial pressure. This will be decided by the neurosurgeon. Another factor here is that the patient may have a bone flap removed, in which case it may not be desirable to turn him onto that side. A compromise may be reached whereby his body is turned as far as possible while his head remains in the supine position. The patient who has had a cerebrovascular accident may have high blood pressure, in which case the head down position will again be contra-indicated.

It may not be possible to put a patient with a flail chest, due to fractured ribs, into side lying and a compromise may again have to be made. By placing pillows under the mattress first at one side and then at the other the patient will be inclined in alternate directions two-hourly. This may apply to the patient with the fractured pelvis, or here he may have his thorax turned one way and then the other while his pelvis remains in the supine position.

87

Patients having peritoneal dialysis may have to remain in one position for the duration of the treatment. During the first few postoperative days the patients in cardiac surgery units may be nursed on a sheepskin in a long-sitting position on a cardiac bed. Patients with diffuse airways obstruction may find it impossible, at least in the early stages, to tolerate some of the postural drainage positions in lying.

If one considers a patient receiving I.P.P.V. through a tracheostomy tube but with no contra-indications preventing accurate postural drainage, the presence of the tubes will not allow it. It is virtually impossible to put the patient into prone lying (though it is possible with a child but it is not a procedure which should be undertaken lightly). Therefore it is very important that collapse of the dorsal segments should be prevented by not allowing the patient to lie on his back at all, at least during the early stages of his illness. He should be nursed in side lying. If it becomes essential to turn the patient into prone, he can be transferred on to a Stryker frame. The frame consists of two canvas stretchers. The patient is lying on pillows on one, for example in the supine position. To turn him into prone more pillows are placed across his body and the second stretcher, with a gap in the canvas for the face, is fixed on top, so that the patient is rather like the meat in a sandwich. A catch is released, the patient taken off the ventilator and the frame rotated 180° round the patient's longitudinal axis. The frame is fixed in position, the patient is attached to the ventilator and the top stretcher and pillows removed. Patients who are on Crutchfield calipers following a high cervical fracture can be nursed on a Stryker frame if necessary.

A respiratory care unit should be equipped with tipping beds which work from a central fulcrum. It should be possible for one person to operate such a bed. In this situation, with the patient in side lying, it will be feasible to position him for the upper zone and the lower zone of each lung and to use the postural drainage positions for the middle lobe and lingula.

The normal two-hourly turning programme which is the rule for the average patient, may be modified to a two and one regime, if indicated by the condition of the chest.

Bearing all the factors of the patient's condition in mind, it must always be the physiotherapist's aim to place him in the most advantageous position to aid chest clearance. The simple fact of moving the patient may have the effect of loosening secretions. If one is not being successful one should make some adjustment to the patient's position.

Manual Technique

Rib springing is a development of one of Lassen's original precepts, that is, squeezing the thorax, which was devised to aid the chest clearance of patients with no ability to breathe or cough due to paralysis. Rib springing should not be used in cases where the chest wall is damaged, for example, fractured ribs; here the physiotherapist's role is supportive. It has proved effective in stimulating a cough and moving secretions in many cases where this is possible, as well as in treating patients who cannot cough. These secretions are then removed by suction.

The physiotherapist places her hands, one on the anterior aspect and one on the posterior aspect of the chest, moulding them to the part. If this is not effective she places her hands, side by side on the chest, with the fingers but not the heels of the hands overlapping. The position of choice will depend upon the size of the patient's thorax and the operator's hands.

Working rhythmically with the ventilator or with the patient's own rate of breathing, the physiotherapist exerts a steadily increasing pressure on the thorax during expiration, ensuring that the whole of the hand is used. There is a tendency to give more pressure with the heel of the hand. This is wrong. Over-pressure is then given at the end of expiration in the form of a short extra push. Care must be taken to ensure that pressure is not relaxed at the end of expiration, that is before over-pressure is given. This faulty technique may cause a fractured rib, especially after repeated application. The use of a piece of sponge rubber between the operator's hands and the patient's chest is particularly valuable for longterm patients whose ribs can become sore after many treatments.

Experiments on rib springing techniques were carried out by Opie and Spalding (1958). They stated: 'Patients being treated by intermittent positive pressure respiration are specially liable to pulmonary complications. In the prophylaxis and treatment of these complications, which may well determine the final outcome, physiotherapy to the chest is of prime importance.' They considered two possible ways in which this technique could act. The first was, that by raising intrathoracic pressure as a whole, air was expelled rapidly from the lungs as in a normal cough and sputum carried along. Their experience indicated that the increase in air flow was insufficient to do this. The second method was by local compression of the consolidated lung, during which secretions were squeezed out, as toothpaste from a tube. This second theory of the way in which rib springing effects chest clearance, was considered to be proven and has been observed on bronchoscopy.

Fine vibrations may be incorporated with rib springing during the expiratory phase and in some cases they are very effective. Vibrations given with slight or even without compression during expiration, are also effective and if done with great care, may aid in the chest clearance of a patient with a damaged chest wall.

Coughing

Effective coughing is the most efficient method of removing secretions from the respiratory system. Under normal conditions, these secretions are moved along by the cilia of the epithelial lining of the bronchial tree, until they reach a point where a cough reflex is stimulated. Coughing is also under voluntary control. It is axiomatic therefore that coughing followed by expectoration is the method of choice for chest clearance.

Many patients requiring intensive respiratory care can cough voluntarily, for example, following cardiac surgery or with diffuse airways obstruction. It will be necessary to support the rib-cage and aid the movement of secretions by positioning and assisted expiration. On occasions supportive pressure over the abdomen will help the patient to cough effectively.

In the majority of conscious patients requiring intensive care voluntary coughing will not be completely successful. The patient will either tire or because of inhibition, due to pain and fear, be unable to clear the chest completely. A suction catheter may be employed either to aspirate secretions from the pharynx or to stimulate a cough reflex which will be followed by aspiration.

Suction catheters may also be used to stimulate a cough reflex in an unconscious patient. If the patient is deeply unconscious it may not be possible to elicit the reflex.

Bag-squeezing is a method of producing maximal expansion of the lungs. It is used in conjunction with positioning and rib springing or simple compression and vibration of the thorax, in an effort to remove secretions by simulating a cough. Bag-squeezing can only be used for patients with either an endotracheal or tracheostomy tube *in situ*. Conscious patients with an endotracheal tube need sedation to enable them to tolerate the tube.

An anaesthetic bag is used and attached to the endotracheal or tracheostomy tube by a short piece of corrugated rubber tubing and a Nosworthy connection.

The bag is taken between both hands and compressed; the aim is maximal expansion of the lungs, so that the bronchi are dilated and air enters the alveoli. A bag of 2 to 4 litres capacity is considered necessary. Inflation should be at a steady rate until maximum expansion is achieved, which is held for a second. Compression of the chest by the physiotherapist starts at this point, so that the peak expiratory flow rate may be used in the effort to simulate a cough. Vibration and compression are continued until expiration is completed. The amount of compression will have to be modified in patients with a damaged chest wall. Accurate timing is essential to achieve the maximum effect. About five or six respirations are given and then the patient is aspirated, unless this is indicated earlier.

The positioning of the patient will be changed during the course of the treatment to ensure clearance of all areas but as usual this will have to be modified in the light of the patient's overall condition.

In many centres the actual bag-squeezing is done by an anaesthetist while the physiotherapist works on the chest, in others the physiotherapist will receive instruction in its use. In either case two people are necessary. Because bag-squeezing can depress cardiac output in patients with poor circulation, many doctors consider that it should be done by either an anaesthetist or a physician. At times a judgement has to be made, as to which is the lesser of the two evils, the patient's lung collapse producing anoxia or depressing cardiac output by the treatment.

Bag-squeezing is also dangerous when used on patients with an air leak from the lung especially where there is a closed chest or clamped drains. In patients with chest drains, these are left unclamped to prevent a tension pneumothorax and to allow any fluid in the pleura to be expressed.

If the patient is being ventilated by a Radcliffe respirator it is possible to give maximum expansion to the patient's lungs by exerting extra pressure on the bellows during the inspiratory phase of the normal respiratory cycle. This method of maximum expansion, used in conjunction with a squeezing of the thorax, has a similar effect to bag-squeezing.

Intermittent positive pressure breathing may be used as a method of aiding chest clearance (see Chapter 3, page 76).

Before, during and after all treatments the physiotherapist is making assessments of the efficacy of her methods and the condition of the patient. In chest work reliance is placed on observation, hearing and the 'feel' of the chest (that is whether there is equal and adequate expansion and the detection of secretions by placing the hand over the area). The use of the stethoscope by physiotherapists is becoming usual practice in many units. Just as with standard physiotherapy methods of assessment, the use of the stethoscope to extend the powers of unaided hearing, which can only detect gross differences from normal breath sounds, requires considerable practice under expert guidance. Some physiotherapists working in chest units and using a stethoscope regularly find its aid invaluable.

MOVEMENT

Some form of movement will be a part of the treatment of a patient requiring intensive care. Occasionally a fully conscious patient will be able to co-operate by doing routine maintenance exercises, others, for example following cardiac surgery, will be able to take part in active assisted movements of their limbs. A percentage of patients in the intensive care unit will either be unconscious or paralysed and therefore will require passive movements. It is not the purpose of this chapter to give detailed instruction in the techniques of passive movements but here are a few points to note.

Particular care should be taken to ensure that full extension of the hips is maintained, by doing this movement in side lying when possible. Some authorities feel that full range abduction of the hip is undesirable in the paraplegic or tetraplegic patient, as this degree of mobility at the hip joints may be a disadvantage to a patient in calipers.

Special attention should be paid to the maintenance of full mobility in the shoulder girdle and glenohumeral joints. These joints seem particularly vulnerable to the development of progressive limitation of movement when the patient is nursed in side lying.

It is possible while maintaining full range joint movement to neglect to produce the full range extensibility in muscles which act over more than one joint. This is particularly so in the long flexors and extensors of the fingers. By passively moving the limbs in the patterns used in facilitation techniques this difficulty can be quickly and easily overcome.

Other points to note, are the importance of maintaining full range passive and accessory movements in the foot and in the hand, particularly the range between the metacarpals. The distance between the thumb and the index finger is another point to consider. The value of the hand as a functioning unit is dramatically diminished if the thumb is fixed in adduction.

In many cases passive movements will be given in side lying as the supine position can be detrimental to the state of the chest.

Problems of spasticity should be treated using one of the many methods available.

For some patients movement may extend beyond the level of maintenance. A progressive exercise programme may be instituted before the patient is able to breathe adequately without a ventilator. Although this situation will not occur often, this aspect of movement should not be overlooked or neglected.

As an adjunct to the maintenance of full range movement, accurate positioning is of great importance for the unconscious or paralysed patient. The positioning of every patient must be considered, but in some cases the patient's general condition will not allow him to be placed in the ideal position from the locomotor point of view. The vast majority of these conscious patients with voluntary movement will recover in a relatively short time and there will be little likelihood of contractures developing.

The unconscious or paralysed patient, who will possibly require prolonged care, will be nursed in side lying and turned two-hourly. It is very important that the patient should remain in the lateral position and not subside into a position 45° to the horizontal. As well as the considerations of chest and pressure areas, the true side-lying position will allow the limbs to be placed accurately. Pillows and sandbags will have the desired effect. One pillow is placed between the patient's back and the mattress and another between the mattress and the frame of the bed. With two pillows so placed the patient cannot roll onto his back. The lower leg is extended and the upper leg is placed on two pillows with the hip and knee flexed about 70°. Both feet are kept at right angles by sandbags or by a combination of pillows and sandbags. The lower shoulder should be adjusted to a comfortable position, usually with the scapula pulled through a little, so that the patient is not actually lying on the point of the shoulder. The upper hand and forearm usually rest on the patient's thigh and the lower one on a pillow, the fingers and wrists are kept in a good position, *i.e.* fingers semiflexed, thumb abducted and wrist extended, by a roll of gamgee tissue. As the patient is turned two-hourly throughout the 24 hours the positioning of the limbs will be reversed at regular intervals.

Spasticity is always a problem and will have to be accommodated in the best way possible.

The positioning of the patient in bed is the joint responsibility of the nursing and physiotherapy staff. Nurses trained in intensive care and neurological work will be aware of the importance of positioning. It is also advisable to seek the assistance of the nursing staff in giving simple passive movements, which should be done at every turn and for the conscious paralysed patient whenever he becomes uncomfortable.

GENERAL NURSING CARE IN WHICH THE PHYSIOTHERAPIST MAY BE INVOLVED

The patient is placed with his head to the foot end of the bed or with the head of the bed removed, to facilitate access to the tracheostomy. There should be ample room for manoeuvre round the patient's head and in some centres, he is placed with his feet towards the wall, as a means of using the space available most advantageously. The patient will be without clothes, which only hinder nursing procedures and may cause pressure sores. The temperature of the room will be sufficient to enable him to be nursed covered only by a sheet. Some patients will dribble from the mouth, in which case the head should be placed either on a rubber sheet covered by paper tissue or on a piece of a paper incontinent sheet which will protect the bed and in either case can easily be changed. Suction of the mouth may be necessary.

The staff must be aware of the dangers of facial palsy, which will prevent the patient from closing the eyes completely or there could be sensory loss affecting the cornea. Irritation, from foreign bodies present in the atmosphere or pressure from the bed linen, may cause corneal ulceration. Tarsorrhaphy (an operative procedure in which the eye is temporarily closed by suturing the lids together) may be used as a protective measure. Micropore or some equivalent adhesive tape may also be used for closure of the eyelids.

Although the general care of the patient is primarily the responsibility of the nursing staff, everyone working in an intensive care unit must be willing to give assistance when necessary and also be very observant of both the patient and the equipment, from the ventilator to the monitor and the intravenous drip.

Turning the patient is a part of physiotherapy treatment and should coincide with the regular turning routine. Speed and efficiency are necessary, especially when turning a patient who is dependent upon a ventilator. Where possible the patient should not be allowed to be supine. It is desirable to have three but essential to have two people to complete the turn of a patient unable to help himself. Having removed as much equipment as possible to the other side of the bed, the operators stand at the side of the bed towards which the patient is facing. The most experienced person takes charge and controls the patient's head and tubes; the second operator stands at hip level and if a third is available she stands opposite to the legs. The pillows are removed and the side-lying position maintained. The operators place their arms as far as possible under the patient's body, pressing down into the mattress to avoid hurting the patient. He is then detached from the ventilator and simultaneously lifted clear of the bed, drawn towards the near side and turned. The patient is immediately re-attached to the ventilator and a pillow placed in his back. Shortly afterwards the patient's chest should be aspirated because of the change of position. The patient's position is adjusted and the pillows replaced. It may be necessary to change the sheets at this time.

Good nursing will prevent the development of pressure sores and such routines as regular turning and lifting the patient clear of the bed during turning, should be adhered to. In one cardiac surgery unit, where for three or four days the patients are nursed in the half-lying position, they are put onto sheepskins. This is very effective in preventing pressure sores.

Many patients will be tube fed, and again physiotherapy treatment involving tipping will need to be timed accordingly, as it is not advisable to tip a patient head down following a feed.

The physiotherapist should be aware of basic nursing techniques and this knowledge should be constantly applied to the general care of the patient and co-operation with the nurses.

TREATMENT

Full details of treatment, for the varied conditions which will require intensive respiratory care, will be covered in the appropriate chapters. The aim at this point is to indicate the way in which the equipment and techniques available to the physiotherapist are utilized in certain basic situations.

As a general rule patients will be treated four-hourly throughout the day, that is 10 a.m., 2 p.m., and 6 p.m., and again at 10 p.m. if necessary. Occasionally a patient will require treatment at intervals throughout the night.

The free-breathing unconscious patient

This may occur in cerebrovascular accident, head injury or following neurosurgery. It may or may not be possible to stimulate a cough reflex. In the simple situation the patients will have normal lungs.

As these patients have disease-free lungs the problems of ensuring good ventilation will not be increased by the presence of excessive secretions. However, it is unlikely that the patient will be breathing deeply ensuring good air entry to all segments of the lungs. Patients may or may not have a tracheostomy.

It is unlikely that the patient will be tipped during treatment, as this may either cause a rise in blood pressure or an increase in intracranial pressure and the state of the chest will not present any serious problems which would make tipping a necessary procedure. He will be nursed in alternate side lying.

If the patient has a cough reflex the most effective method of moving secretions will be to stimulate a cough. This can be done in two ways, either by rib springing and vibrations or by using a suction catheter, which will then be in a position to aspirate. A combination of these methods is very effective. As well as assisting in chest clearance, rib springing or simple thoracic compression during expiration will increase the depth of respiration and improve the ventilation of the lungs.

The patient will first be treated on one side and then turned to the opposite side to complete chest clearance. If the physiotherapist detects the presence of secretions which are not responding to simple side lying and coughing, the positioning of the patient should be adapted as far as possible to the standard postural drainage position for the area.

If the patient is so deeply unconscious that a cough reflex cannot be stimulated, the physiotherapist will have to rely on the squeezing effect of rib springing. In this case, aspiration without an endotracheal or tracheostomy tube will be relatively ineffective, as the secretions will remain in the trachea and the possibility of the suction catheter reaching this level via the nose or mouth is debatable. Such a patient is liable to develop a chest infection and/or segmental or lung collapse.

Patients who have either an endotracheal or a tracheostomy tube *in situ* will need humidification.

Full range passive movements will be given.

The free-breathing conscious patient who is able to co-operate

He will usually require a certain percentage of oxygen and therefore he will be wearing a face mask or nasal spectacles.

There are essentially two types of patient in this group: the first is in the early post-operative period, some following cardiac surgery, and the second has diffuse airways obstruction. Both types of patient will require humidification because they are breathing a percentage of dry gas but the patient with chronic lung disease is likely to have copious sticky sputum, the removal of which will be assisted by humidification incorporating a mucolytic agent, or bronchial spasm which may respond to a bronchodilatory drug.

All these patients will be able to co-operate by coughing but it is unlikely that their efforts will be effective enough to ensure adequate chest clearance.

In one centre, following cardiac surgery, the patient is nursed in the half-lying position and in the very early stages he will not be moved as a means of aiding chest clearance. Patients will be in some pain, with a large incision, chest drains and a drip and will be wired for monitoring. The first method of chest clearance is breathing followed by assisted coughing. The physiotherapist will assist the patient by using gentle pressure with vibrations during expiration, either over the ribs or sternum. At a suitable point the physiotherapist will stabilize the chest while the patient coughs. After some time the patient may tire and may not be able to get the sputum beyond the pharynx. At this point nasal suction is indicated. Following good pre-operative preparation the vast majority of patients are remarkably co-operative.

At times, either due to fatigue or inhibited by fear, the patient will not be able to cough. It will then be necessary to use the catheter as a means of stimulating a cough reflex as well as for aspiration.

The chest X-rays will always be available and should be studied prior to treatment.

Assisted active exercises will follow chest clearance.

The patient with chronic lung disease may be reluctant to take up a position to aid chest clearance but with explanation and persuasion he will usually co-operate.

Treatment is frequently preceded by a short period on the ultrasonic nebulizer; occasionally a patient will be on a nebulizer for a prolonged period. As the patient has an intact chest wall, rib springing, vibrations and shaking will be used to move secretions. The patient's efforts may be ineffective and suction will be necessary to assist him.

Intermittent positive pressure breathing is used in some centres and is found to be of benefit to all patients in this group as a means of gaining adequate lung expansion and as a means of assisted coughing (see Chapter 3, page 76 *et seq.*).

A very small percentage of conscious patients with varying conditions will be found to be unable or unwilling to cough effectively and therefore reflex coughing and suction will be necessary.

A patient with a damaged chest wall, some ability to breathe but requiring I.P.P.V. to ensure adequate respiration

The typical patient will have fractured ribs.

Fractures of the ribs usually occur near to the angle and in the majority of cases are caused by direct violence.

The fracture of one or two ribs will be very painful and the patient will be unwilling either to breathe deeply or cough effectively. Breathing exercises and assisted coughing will be all that the patient requires.

Patients with moderate chest injuries cannot cough adequately and maintain a clear airway. It may be necessary to insert a tracheostomy tube and aspirate. If the cuff is inflated inhalation of foreign matter will be prevented. This is of particular importance if the patient is unconscious.

In severe chest injury where there are multiple fractures, especially if both sides of the rib-cage are involved, the anterior part of the chest wall will be flail. Paradoxical breathing will occur, *i.e.* in inspiration the relatively damaged part of the chest wall will be drawn in. The reverse will happen on expiration. There is also a shunting to and fro of air in adjacent bronchi, which results in the loss of a larger area of effective lung than that directly affected by the injury.

The ventilation of the lungs is seriously impaired by this situation, added to which the airway may be obstructed by blood, and blood and air will have entered the pleural cavity. The patient, if conscious, will be in great pain.

To ensure a clear airway and adequate ventilation the patient will have been given a tracheostomy and placed on I.P.P.V. I.P.P.V. also acts as a form of internal splintage and prevents paradoxical breathing. It is probable that the patient will be placed on a self-triggering ventilator. Ventilation will be continued for 10 to 14 days or until the ribs stabilize.

This type of injury is frequently referred to as a 'stove-in chest'.

If the chest is flail the patient will have a chest drain and it is possible that he will have other injuries.

Positioning to aid drainage of the lungs will be very restricted if it is possible at all. It may simply consist of inclining the patient first to one side and then to the other by placing pillows between the mattress and the bed frame.

It is obvious that direct pressure on the damaged part of the thorax in this situation cannot be contemplated. Bag-squeezing can be helpful in loosening secretions.

Suction will be necessary to remove the blood and secretions from the trachea. Many of these patients are conscious and the vast majority have a cough reflex which will be stimulated by the suction catheter. Coughing will be extremely painful and the physiotherapist should use her hands to stabilize the rib-cage while the nurse aspirates.

Active assisted movements will be given where and when indicated.

Patients with diseased lungs and difficulty in maintaining a clear airway and adequate ventilation but with an undamaged chest wall and some ability to breathe spontaneously

This type of patient usually has an acute exacerbation of his diffuse airways obstruction.

As the patient will attempt to breathe he may be nursed on a self-triggering ventilator. A mixture of air and 40% oxygen is frequently given and drugs, such as bronchodilators or mucolytic agents, may be added to the humidifying system.

If artificial ventilation is expected to be of short duration an endotracheal tube may be used but for prolonged ventilation the patient will need a tracheostomy.

All the usual methods of chest clearance may be used to remove the copious quantities of sputum. There is unlikely to be any contraindication to tipping and the intact chest wall allows rib springing to be used, although this may be difficult in patients with overinflated chests. Vibrations may be easier and more effective. Suction will be given at frequent intervals and reflex coughing may be stimulated.

The number of treatments given in the 24 hours will be dictated by the condition of the patient but it must not be forgotten that he will need some rest.

The patient will be encouraged to do simple maintenance exercises.

The patient has paralysis of the muscles of respiration with complete or partial incompetence of swallowing and gross or complete general paralysis

This may occur in polyneuritis, myasthenia gravis, drug overdose and tetanus.

(In severe cases of tetanus, death from asphyxia due to spasm of the respiratory and laryngeal muscles or from the inspiration of secretions was common. The use of the paralysing drug curare to control the spasm in conjunction with I.P.P.V. has proved to be a most successful form of treatment. Death occasionally occurs and in some cases this is thought to be due to the effects of tetanus toxin on the brain stem.)

Patients with polyneuritis, myasthenia gravis and tetanus are completely conscious. This is sometimes difficult to remember with any patient who is totally paralysed as he will appear to be unconscious. It is very easy to talk over such a patient, entirely forgetting that he will be able to hear what is being said. Even patients whom we believe to be unconscious may not be totally unaware when staff are speaking near by, even if they are unable to respond. It is obvious that great care should be exercised when talking to a colleague close to such patients and one should make a point of talking to the patient and explaining what is happening, if there is any possibility that he might understand.

Patients in this group are in a similar position to the patients with anterior poliomyelitis, to whose plight Dr. Lassen responded by developing a method of positive pressure ventilation via a cuffed tracheostomy tube.

A well-tried treatment routine starts with the patient in the side-lying position in which the physiotherapist finds him when she enters the ward. The patient is tipped head up in a position for drainage of the upper zone. The physiotherapist, working if possible with a nurse, who will help by aspirating the patient and assisting with turning, starts rib springing. If no secretions are moved within about 10 minutes and the physiotherapist feels that the area is not clear some adjustment to the patient's position is indicated.

If the area is clear the bed will be tipped in the opposite direction to drain the lower zone and rib springing continued. Suction is given when secretions are detected and before and after a change of position.

Following clearance of the lower zone it may be necessary to position the patient for drainage of the middle lobe or lingula.

When that side of the chest is clear, the bed will be returned to the horizontal and some of the pillows and sandbags removed to allow full range passive movements of the uppermost limbs to be given with the patient still in side lying. The patient is then turned and aspirated as soon as possible following a period of ventilation. Passive movements to the second side are given, the pillows replaced and the patient made comfortable.

The chest clearance pattern is then repeated for the second time. The cuff should be released with the patient in the head down position. With the head lowered, secretions released from round the cuff and present in the mouth and pharynx cannot enter the lungs. If the cuff is not let down four-hourly it may not coincide with physiotherapy. This is the moment when the patient can speak, as air passes over the vocal cords. The cuff is reinflated and the patient returned to the horizontal.

WEANING FROM A VENTILATOR

As the patient begins to recover his respiratory function he is disconnected from the ventilator for a short time. Free breathing is easier after chest clearance and before general exercises. As the movement programme will be progressing, it is advisable to practise breathing before the patient tires. Regular short spells of free breathing are advisable.

Some patients will be apprehensive and on no account should the ventilator be switched off, as its noisy presence is very reassuring.

No patient should be encouraged to breathe beyond his own limit; if this happens he may become exhausted and under-ventilated or he may be afraid next time free breathing is suggested.

If by chance the patient has been over-ventilated mechanically he will be accustomed to a low PCO_2 and he will find free breathing difficult. This is corrected by gradually reducing the mechanical ventilation.

Most patients find it easier to breathe in supine lying with a pillow under the knees. By placing her hands on either side of the chest wall the physiotherapist facilitates movement. If necessary a free breathing chart may be kept to demonstrate the patient's progress.

The inflated cuff prevents air from escaping round the tube and it is thought that it is easier to breathe with the cuff inflated rather than with it deflated. Some authorities have cast doubt on this view. This may be followed by placing a cork in the tracheostomy tube after deflating the cuff, which brings the dead air space into the respiratory system. When assisted ventilation is no longer necessary the tube is changed and a silver one inserted. Finally the tracheostome is sealed with a dressing and in most cases it heals naturally. Sometimes plastic surgery is necessary and this gives a better cosmetic effect.

Swallowing may return spontaneously but with some cases of myasthenia gravis complete control is never regained. In one particularly severe case the patient was eventually fed with liquidized food through a tube directly into the stomach.

REFERENCES AND BIBLIOGRAPHY

Chamney, Anne R. (1969). 'Humidification requirements and techniques.' *Anaesthesia*, Vol. 24, No. 4.

Clement, A. J. & Hubsch, S. K. (1968). *Physiotherapy*, **54**, 355.

Gardner, E. K. & Shelton, Brenda (1967). *The Intensive Therapy Unit and the Nurse*. Faber & Faber Ltd., London.

Gaskell, Diana (1970). 'The Bird Mark 7 Ventilator.' *Physiotherapy*, **56**, 360.

Gilston, A. & Resnekov, L. (1971). *Cardio-Respiratory Resuscitation*. Heinemann Medical Books Ltd., London.

Myles, P. V. (1970). 'Use of the Entonox Machine in Post-operative Chest Surgery.' *Physiotherapy*, **56**, 559.

Norris, Walter & Campbell, Donald (1971). *Anaesthetics, Resuscitation and Intensive Care—A textbook for students and residents.* Churchill-Livingstone, Edinburgh. 3rd ed.

Sara, C. (1965). 'The Management of Patients with a Tracheostomy.' *Med. J. Aust.,* **1**, 99.

Spalding, J. M. K. & Crampton Smith, A. *Clinical Practice and Physiology of Artificial Respiration.* Blackwell Scientific Publications, Oxford.

Stramin, L., Abrams, M. E. & Simpson, B. R. (1968). 'Effects of Bronchial Lavage on Pulmonary Surfactant.' *Proc. R. Soc. Med.,* **61**, 1162.

Waddington, P. J. (1969). *Physiotherapy in Artificial Respiration.* Churchill-Livingstone, Edinburgh.

CHAPTER 5

Introduction to the Treatment of Medical Chest Conditions

by D. V. GASKELL, M.C.S.P.

Before undertaking the treatment of chest conditions it is important for the physiotherapy student to be familiar with the main signs and symptoms of respiratory disease. A more experienced physiotherapist should also have some knowledge of reading X-rays, be able to use a stethoscope and be able to interpret the results of lung function tests and blood gas analysis, but it is beyond the scope of this chapter to cover these more specialized skills.

COMMON CLINICAL MANIFESTATIONS IN RESPIRATORY DISEASE

Cough

Coughing is a forced expiration against a closed glottis. A high pressure of air is built up in the trachea and major airways and the sudden opening of the glottis is followed by an explosive discharge producing the characteristic noise. It is one of the commonest signs of respiratory disease and will be stimulated by the presence of excessive secretions in the respiratory tract or by other irritations of the nerve endings in the larynx, trachea, bronchi or even the pleura. Many smokers regard a morning cough as normal.

Sputum

The normal adult forms about 100 ml of mucus from his respiratory tract daily. This blanket of mucus is removed by the action of the

104

cilia which beat upwards in the direction of the larynx, and carries with it any small particles of dust etc. deposited on the mucosal lining of the lung. Excess mucus, or failure of the normal process of removal, will stimulate the cough reflex and mucus will be expectorated as sputum.

Sputum may be mucoid, black or grey, blood-stained or contain plugs or casts. *Mucoid* sputum is clear or white. Black or grey sputum may be mucoid but flecked with black or grey deposit due to various causes such as cigarette smoke, atmospheric pollution, coal dust etc. *Purulent* sputum may contain a variable amount of pus, it is usually yellow, but may become green and foul-smelling. If there is only a small amount of pus present, sputum is described as *mucopurulent*.

Blood-stained sputum varies from slight streaking to gross haemoptysis when the patient coughs pure blood. Blood-stained sputum must always be reported to the physician in charge of the patient and should always be investigated. It occurs in bronchiectasis and in some cases of simple bronchitis but it may be an early sign of carcinoma or pulmonary tuberculosis. *Rusty* blood-stained sputum is a feature of lobar pneumonia.

Plugs and casts may be found in the sputum of patients with pulmonary eosinophilia as in asthma, aspergillosis, farmer's lung etc.

It is very important for the physiotherapist to observe the type of sputum expectorated by the patient and to note any change in its appearance or quantity.

Some patients have particularly thick and viscid sputum, which is often noticeable in the early stages of an infection when the patient has a fever and may be slightly dehydrated. Care should be taken not to nurse the patient in a dry atmosphere, the intake of fluid should be encouraged and if oxygen is being given it should be humidified. Thick secretions can also be moistened by extra humidification, which can range from simple steam inhalations to the use of ultrasonic nebulizers. If intermittent humidification is being given, it is helpful if the physiotherapist can treat the patient immediately afterwards.

Dyspnoea

This is an awareness of difficulty in breathing which may be due to a variety of causes. It may vary considerably in degree. After exercise normal healthy people may have rapid breathing (tachypnoea) and experience mild transient dyspnoea which may not be distressing. Dyspnoea can be observed in patients suffering from severe emphysema. Breathlessness precipitated by lying flat and relieved by sitting up is known as *orthopnoea*.

Wheeze

This is a musical sound mainly heard on *expiration* and caused by *airways obstruction*. Airways obstruction may be caused by narrowing of the bronchial lumen due to bronchospasm, oedema of the bronchial mucosa or excessive secretions; it is the combination of these factors together with the normal shortening and narrowing of the bronchus on expiration which causes the wheeze. A typical wheeze can be heard in asthmatic patients. More rarely a wheeze may be caused by bronchial stenosis or a foreign body.

A wheeze can be greatly exaggerated if the patient forces his expiration.

Stridor

This is a musical sound mainly heard on *inspiration* and is caused by obstruction in the trachea or larynx.

Chest Pain

This is frequently due to pleuritic pain which is sharp and stabbing in character and worse on coughing or deep breathing when the patient may 'catch' his breath. It is usually localized but may be referred to the abdominal wall, or with diaphragmatic pleurisy to the tip of the shoulder. There are many other causes of chest pain such as fractured ribs, intercostal nerve root pain, costochondritis, intrathoracic neoplasms, coronary insufficiency (see page 274) and others. If in doubt as to the cause of chest pain, the physiotherapist should always discuss the matter with the physician before carrying on with the treatment.

Cyanosis

This means 'blueness'. It is caused by *hypoxaemia* (lack of oxygen) and is not always easy to judge unless it is severe. Cyanosis may also be associated with *hypercapnia* (increased carbon dioxide concentration in arterial blood).

Finger Clubbing

This is the filling in of the angle between the skin and the base of the nail. Later there is increased curvature of the nails and the pulps of the fingers become enlarged.

In pulmonary disease this is usually associated with chronic septic conditions such as lung abscess, severe bronchiectasis, cystic fibrosis or with neoplasm. It may also be associated with other diseases or may be familial with no underlying cause.

DIAGNOSTIC PROCEDURES

Radiography

Examination of postero-anterior and lateral chest films will be carried out and compared with any previous X-rays. If necessary the physician may order *tomography* when films taken of the lungs are focussed at different depths, or *fluoroscopy* or *screening* which allows examination of the heart, lungs and diaphragm in the dynamic state. A *bronchogram* may be performed. This is the introduction of opaque iodized oil into the bronchi which outlines the bronchial tree and may reveal bronchiectasis (see page 143). Various other investigations such as a barium meal may also be ordered.

Examination of Bronchial Secretions

Sputum examination is of great value in the diagnosis and treatment of chest disease. Pathological investigation of the sputum may include microscopic examination for malignant cells or bacteria, culture for identification of bacteria and determination of their sensitivity to antibiotics.

Diagnostic Skin Tests

These will include tuberculin testing and allergy reactions (see page 148).

Bronchoscopy

This is direct visualization of the bronchial tree through a tube passed down the throat between the vocal cords under local or general anaesthesia. Vision is possible as far as the segmental bronchi. It is a valuable diagnostic procedure and provides a means of taking bronchial biopsies.

It may also be required for removal of secretions if the patient is unable to cough them up himself or for removal of a foreign body lodged in the airways. In these situations it is important for the physiotherapist to treat the patient as soon as he has recovered from the anaesthetic. Postural drainage with effective coughing and breathing exercises should be carried out.

Pulmonary Function Studies

These will give much valuable information (see Chapter 2, page 40).

Pleural and Lung Biopsy

These are carried out via thoracoscopy or small thoracotomy incisions (see Chapter 9, page 187).

Definition of Types of Disease

OBSTRUCTIVE AIRWAYS DISEASE

The flow of air through the lungs may be reduced by obstruction in the airways. Common causes of this are excessive secretions, broncho-spasm, or oedema of the bronchial mucosa. Frequently a combination of all three is found, as in acute asthmatic attacks.

Airways obstruction may also be the result of scar tissue narrowing or kinking the bronchi, as can happen in chronic bronchitis, or it may follow the destruction of the elastic honeycomb structure of the lung as in some cases of emphysema. The bronchi lose the support of the surrounding lung and tend to collapse in expiration.

Air flow through the bronchi can be assessed by measurement of *peak expiratory flow* (using the Wright Peak Flow Meter) or the F.E.V.$_1$ (*forced expiratory volume in 1 second*) which is normally 70–80% of the F.V.C. (*forced vital capacity*).

Reversible Airways Obstruction

In some cases F.E.V.$_1$ and peak flow measurements improve after the patient is given a bronchodilator (*e.g.* salbutamol, isoprenaline). Reversibility of airways obstruction is a hopeful sign; a bronchodilator or steroid regime may overcome bronchospasm and give relief.

Such cases often have mucus hypersecretion and respond well to appropriate physiotherapy. Asthma and early chronic bronchitis are diseases in which airways obstruction is usually reversible.

Irreversible or Fixed Airways Obstruction

Irreversibility is demonstrated when administration of a bronchodilator fails to secure any improvement in the peak flow or F.E.V.$_1$. This shows that the airways have suffered structural damage; little improvement can be expected from drugs, and physiotherapy is directed towards improving the efficiency of respiration in the face of the defect.

Severe chronic bronchitis, generalized bronchiectasis, and severe emphysema provide examples of this condition. A degree of reversibility may be found superimposed on a fixed obstructive defect. Alleviation of the reversible element may bring about improvement and is always worth trying.

RESTRICTIVE PULMONARY DISEASE

Air flow in the lungs may be hindered in the absence of any bronchial disease. Ankylosing spondylitis or kyphoscoliosis may cause abnormalities of the rib-cage which restrict expansion of the lung. Restrictive defects may also be caused by diffuse interstitial pulmonary fibrosis (fibrosing alveolitis), pleural fibrosis, widespread post-tuberculous fibrosis and pulmonary oedema. In this latter group of conditions, it is a change in pulmonary compliance (stiffness) that restricts the expansion of the lung.

Patients with restrictive lung disease may need to breathe more rapidly (tachypnoea) to satisfy their respiratory needs, because the lung volumes are reduced and they cannot take deep breaths. Diseases of the lung itself often interfere with the alveolar wall, adding difficulties of gas transfer to those of pulmonary restriction.

RESPIRATORY FAILURE

When the lungs cannot maintain an adequate gas exchange respiratory failure is said to exist. Campbell has suggested that a PO_2 below 60 mm Hg at rest or a PCO_2 above 49 mm Hg should be used to define respiratory failure.

It may be caused by depression of the respiratory centre by poisons, drugs, anoxia, head injuries, or cerebral disease; by failure of the respiratory muscles as in poliomyelitis, acute polyneuritis and myasthenia gravis; by loss of functioning lung tissue as in extensive pneumonia, pulmonary collapse, pneumothorax, following resection of lung tissue, or crush injury of the chest wall; by obstructive airways disease as in status asthmaticus or in acute exacerbations of chronic bronchitis. Patients with chronic lung disease are particularly prone to respiratory failure.

The aims of the treatment are to maintain clear airways and to ensure adequate alveolar ventilation whilst treating the underlying cause. If the failure is associated with a normal or low PCO_2, oxygen therapy will not present any problems, but if the patient is in *hypercapnic respiratory failure* with a low PO_2 and a high PCO_2, oxygen therapy must be very carefully controlled as the free use of oxygen may remove the patient's only remaining ventilatory drive. A safe method of giving controlled oxygen is by means of a Ventimask (see Fig. 3/4, page 66). There are three types which supply 24%, 28% or 35% concentrations of oxygen respectively.

Physiotherapy has a vital role to play in the removal of secretions and the maintenance of adequate ventilation, by means of postural drainage, effective coughing and deep breathing.

It may be necessary to consider some form of assisted ventilation either by means of I.P.P.B. (intermittent positive pressure breathing) or by intubation and artificial ventilation. Some patients may require a tracheostomy but many physicians are reluctant to consider this when the patient has a long history of chronic lung disease.

COR PULMONALE

In 1961 the World Health Organization offered the following definition of cor pulmonale:

'Hypertrophy of the right ventricle resulting from diseases affecting the function and/or the structure of the lung, except when these pulmonary alterations are the result of diseases that primarily affect the left side of the heart or of congenital heart disease.'

Cor pulmonale most commonly occurs in association with longstanding pulmonary disease such as chronic bronchitis, bronchiectasis or with diffuse fibrosis of the lungs following pneumoconiosis etc. It may be seen in longstanding kyphoscoliosis and also following obstruction of the pulmonary vascular bed by pulmonary emboli. It is rarely seen in primary emphysema.

It is frequently precipitated by a respiratory infection causing hypoxia and carbon dioxide retention superimposed upon chronic pulmonary disease. Initially CO_2 retention produces an increase in cardiac output and systemic arteriolar dilatation resulting in a bounding pulse.

Dilatation of cerebral vessels may produce headache, raised intracranial pressure and papilloedema. The pulmonary arterioles constrict in response to hypoxia; this effect combines with the increased cardiac output to produce pulmonary hypertension which may be further aggravated if many of the pulmonary blood vessels are obliterated by disease. In the later stages of the disease pulmonary hypertension becomes severe (reaching systemic levels) and right ventricular failure develops as a result of the enormous work load and continuing hypoxia.

Clinical Features

In addition to signs of the original disease, the patient is cyanosed, the extremities warm and the pulse full. The jugular venous pressure is raised, the liver enlarged and dependent oedema will be present. An electrocardiogram may show the large, sharply pointed P-waves of right atrial hypertrophy and there may be signs of right ventricular hypertrophy. As the cardiac output falls, the extremities become cold and the pulse small; venous congestion and oedema increase. The chest X-ray reveals cardiac enlargement and dilatation of the main pulmonary arteries.

Treatment

The main aim of treatment is to improve the alveolar ventilation. This will be by means of bronchodilators, oxygen therapy, physio-

111

therapy and antibiotics. Diuretics with potassium supplements will be given for the cardiac failure. Digitalis therapy is seldom of great use. Once the underlying pulmonary condition starts to respond to treatment, the cardiac condition will improve.

PHYSIOTHERAPY

Treatment should be vigorous and aimed at clearing the airways of excess secretions and improving alveolar ventilation. I.P.P.B. is often helpful as many patients are slightly confused and unable to co-operate fully. Some patients tolerate postural drainage well but if the patient becomes cyanosed and distressed during this procedure, they may be more comfortable in a modified position. Oxygen therapy should be continued during physiotherapy and the mask only removed when the patient wishes to expectorate.

Treatments should be short and frequent; care should be taken not to tire the patient.

Ideally treatment should be carried out for about 20 minutes every two hours for the first 48 hours. If persistent hypoxaemia, hypercapnia and acidosis are shown on arterial blood gas analysis, the patient should be roused, given I.P.P.B., and encouraged to cough at intervals during the night.

When the patient's condition improves, treatments can be cut down and continued along the lines for the original disease.

CLINICAL ASSESSMENT OF THE CHEST

The physician will examine the patient's chest by means of inspection, palpation, percussion and auscultation. A physiotherapist experienced in chest work may like to repeat this examination at intervals during the course of treatment but it is not always possible to teach physiotherapy students accurate use of the stethoscope during their training. However, the student can obtain a great deal of information by reading the doctor's notes, looking at the X-rays, questioning the patient and also by general observation of the patient.

Inspection

The patient's pattern of breathing should be observed. Many patients have a characteristic pattern. In asthma, chronic bronchitis and emphysema they may have an over-inflated chest and most of the respiratory movements occur in the apical region; they may even have paradoxical movement of the lower ribs. An abdominal 'bounce', due to a sudden increase in obstruction, may be present in severe emphysematous patients (see page 162); these patients may also breathe out with 'pursed lips'. It has been suggested that the resultant back pressure may prevent collapse of airways and subsequent air-trapping. Many patients use the accessory muscles, varying from a slight contraction of the sternomastoids to the use of trapezius and elevation of the shoulder girdle with every inspiratory effort.

The rate of respiration should be observed as the patient may be noted to be dyspnoeic either at rest or after the effort of undressing. Note of cyanosis or clubbing should also be made.

Palpation

Any chest deformities should be observed and a physiotherapist may often note decreased movement by placing her hands on either side of the thorax and asking the patient to take a deep breath.

It is sometimes helpful to take chest measurements. The resting measurement should be recorded, followed by full expiration and full inspiration. The measurements should be taken at three levels, at the fourth costal cartilage, at the level of the xiphoid process, and at the level of the ninth costal cartilage. This will often reveal an over-inflated upper chest with poor basal movement, particularly in asthma, chronic bronchitis, and emphysema. If a peak flow meter or vitalograph are available, it is helpful to measure the peak flow or F.E.V.$_1$ before and after physiotherapy.

PHYSIOTHERAPY IN THE TREATMENT OF MEDICAL CHEST CONDITIONS

Postural Drainage

Postural drainage consists of placing the patient in various positions designed to drain secretions from the different segments of the lungs by means of gravity. This can be further assisted by vibrations or shaking on expiration and clapping over the chest wall. Postural drainage will drain secretions from the periphery of the lung to the larger airways, from where they can be coughed up more easily.

The length of time spent in each position will vary from patient to patient and will depend on the type and quantity of sputum being expectorated. Each individual patient must be carefully considered, X-rays must be studied and if a bronchogram is available it is of considerable help when working out postural drainage positions.

It may be necessary to spend an average of 15 to 20 minutes in each position and occasionally even longer. Ideally the patient should remain in each position until that particular area has been cleared, which may necessitate draining different areas at alternate treatments. The most badly affected area should always be drained first. Postural drainage should never be carried out immediately after a meal.

If a patient has reversible airways obstruction, it is often helpful to give a bronchodilator about 15 minutes before postural drainage, as coughing can aggravate bronchospasm particularly in asthmatic patients. If secretions are very thick and tenacious, a mist or steam inhalation may be given beforehand.

During postural drainage the patient should be encouraged to take deep breaths and to cough at intervals. By this means, the collateral airdrift between the alveoli can be made use of in order to remove secretions from smaller airways. The patient should remain clothed during treatment as percussion over the bare chest wall is painful. Any tight or extra warm clothing should obviously be removed.

POSTURAL DRAINAGE POSITIONS

Upper Lobe

1. APICAL BRONCHUS (Fig. 5/1)
The patient should sit upright, with slight variations according to the position of the lesion which may necessitate leaning slightly backwards, forwards or sideways. This position is usually only necessary for infants or patients being nursed in a recumbent position, but occasionally may be required if there is an abscess or stenosis of a bronchus in the apical region.

2. POSTERIOR BRONCHUS
   (a) *Right* (Fig. 5/2)
The patient should lie on his left side horizontally, and then turn 45°

114

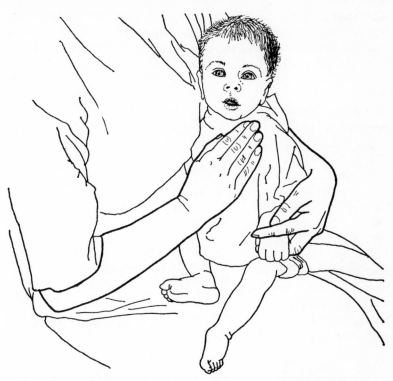

FIG. 5/1. Postural drainage position for the apical segment, left upper lobe

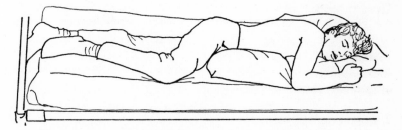

FIG. 5/2. Postural drainage position for the posterior segment, right upper lobe

on to his face, resting against a pillow with another supporting his head.

(*b*) *Left* (Fig. 5/3)

The patient should lie on his right side turned 45° onto his face with 3 pillows arranged to raise the shoulders 12 inches (30 cm) from the bed.

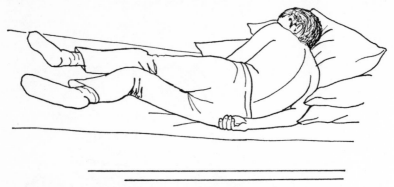

FIG. 5/3. Postural drainage position for the posterior segment, left upper lobe

3. ANTERIOR BRONCHUS (Fig. 5/4)

The patient should lie flat on his back with his knees slightly flexed.

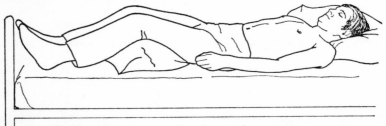

FIG. 5/4. Postural drainage position for anterior segments, upper lobe

Middle Lobe

4. LATERAL BRONCHUS

5. MEDIAL BRONCHUS

The patient should lie flat on his back with his body quarter turned to the left maintained by a pillow under the right side from shoulder

116

to hip. The foot of the bed should be raised 14 inches (35 cm) from the ground (Fig. 5/5).

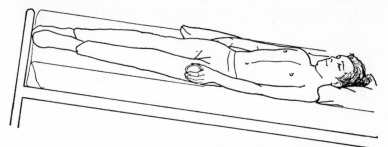

FIG. 5/5. Postural drainage position for the right middle lobe

Lingula

6. SUPERIOR BRONCHUS

7. INFERIOR BRONCHUS
The patient should lie flat on his back with his body quarter turned to the right maintained by a pillow under the left side from shoulder to hip.

The foot of the bed should be raised 14 inches (35 cm) from the ground.

Lower Lobe

8. APICAL BRONCHUS (Fig. 5/6)
The patient should lie flat on his face with a pillow under his hips.

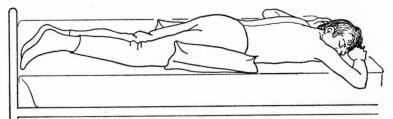

FIG. 5/6. Postural drainage position for the apical segments, lower lobes

9. MEDIAL BASAL (CARDIAC) BRONCHUS (Fig. 5/7)

The patient should lie on his right side with a pillow under his hips and foot of bed should be raised 18 inches (46 cm) from the ground.

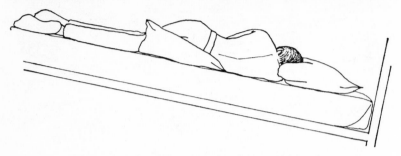

FIG. 5/7. Postural drainage position for right medial basal segment and left lateral basal segment

10. ANTERIOR BASAL BRONCHUS (Fig. 5/8)

The patient should lie flat on his back, the buttocks resting on a pillow and the knees bent, the foot of the bed should be raised 18 inches (46 cm) from the ground.

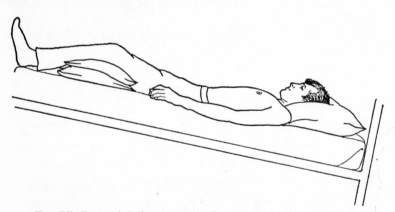

FIG. 5/8. Postural drainage position for the anterior basal segments

11. LATERAL BASAL BRONCHUS (Fig. 5/9)

The patient should lie on the opposite side, the foot of the bed should be raised 18 inches (46 cm) from the ground. It is helpful to place an extra pillow under the patient's hips.

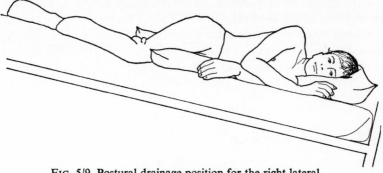

FIG. 5/9. Postural drainage position for the right lateral
basal segment

12. POSTERIOR BASAL BRONCHUS (Fig. 5/10)
The patient should lie flat on his face with a pillow under the hips,
the foot of the bed should be raised 18 inches (46 cm) from the
ground.

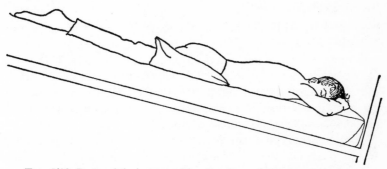

FIG. 5/10. Postural drainage position for the posterior basal segments

Inhalations Given in Association with Postural Drainage

Bronchodilators, steam inhalations, mist therapy and mucolytic
agents should always be given *before* postural drainage. Inhalations
of antibiotics or antifungal agents should be given *after* postural
drainage.

Bronchography

Before a bronchogram the patient should be given postural drainage if there appear to be excessive secretions which would prevent adequate filling of the bronchi.

After a bronchogram patients with bronchiectasis or cystic fibrosis should be given postural drainage in order to clear the radio-opaque medium from the bronchi; in other conditions some will be removed by the action of the cilia, the rest will be absorbed by the blood stream.

Modified Postural Drainage

Certain patients may be too dyspnoeic to tolerate postural drainage, particularly those with severe bronchospasm or emphysema. It is better to turn this type of patient onto alternate sides for short periods of time without tipping the bed. Some will tolerate lying flat, others prefer to be propped up with several pillows. Shaking, vibrations and clapping may be given in this position.

Postural Drainage at Home

Many patients with chronic chest disease will need to carry out postural drainage at home. This can often present problems as it may be necessary to tip the bed and this is not always possible. This problem can be overcome by placing a 6 inch (15 cm) thick pile of newspapers or magazines tied tightly together on the bed and placing pillows on top of this. The patient can lie over this in varying positions and thus drain most areas of his lungs.

Young patients can drain the posterior basal areas by lying over the side of the bed with their forearms resting on the floor, but this position cannot be maintained for any length of time.

Babies and small children can be given postural drainage over their mother's knee.

Before a patient is discharged from hospital the physiotherapist should instruct him in how to carry out postural drainage at home adapting to the various situations. The timing factor should be taken into consideration as it is not always possible to spend as long on drainage in the home. The patient should be encouraged to spend as long as is practical until the worst of the secretions have been cleared, *e.g.* 15 to 20 minutes, possibly less.

Contra-indications to Postural Drainage

1. Recent haemoptysis. Once the bleeding has stopped, postural drainage may usually be resumed but permission should always be sought from the physician first. It is better not to percuss for a day or so.
2. Severe hypertension.
3. Certain cardiac arrythmias.
4. Following recent head injuries.
5. If there is regurgitation of gastric juices as in hiatus hernia.
6. Tension pneumothorax.
7. Severe surgical emphysema.
8. Aneurysm or obstruction of main blood vessels.
9. Pulmonary oedema.

BREATHING CONTROL

The term 'Breathing Exercises' is misleading as it implies that the patient is physically exerting himself. In fact, many patients suffering from respiratory disease are already expending far too much effort on respiration and need to be taught how to control their breathing, hence the title of this controversial section.

There are several different techniques of teaching breathing control and there is still some controversy about the precise action of certain respiratory muscles and about the mechanics of breathing (Campbell, Agostoni & Newsom Davis, 1970). Physiotherapists must be prepared to change the rationale of their techniques as more experiments are performed in this field. They must also be prepared for disappointing results of certain lung function tests before and after treatment. Although the patient with emphysema may have obviously improved and his exercise tolerance increased, the $F.E.V._1$ may remain disappointingly low; on the other hand, this type of patient will show improvement in his respiratory pressure volume relationship (Innocenti, 1966). Patients with asthma will often show improvement in their $F.E.V._1$ after effective treatment. As more sophisticated lung function tests are developed, it is to be hoped that the effects of breathing control will be more fully understood.

121

Diaphragmatic Breathing

The diaphragm is the main respiratory muscle and the student must have a thorough knowledge of its action before attempting to teach this technique to patients.

One method of teaching diaphragmatic breathing concentrates on forward movement of the whole abdominal wall. A second technique, advocated by the writer, combines forward movement of the upper abdominal wall with some lateral movement of the lower ribs.

POSITION OF THE PATIENT

Diaphragmatic breathing is usually taught in a half-lying or sitting position, particularly if the patient is short of breath due to chest disease. In the supine position the domes of the diaphragm will be elevated due to the weight of abdominal viscera and this may be distressing to patients suffering from dyspnoea.

When treating the majority of cases, the patient should be well-supported with pillows or cushions and should be sitting straight, the iliac crests should be level as faulty posture could cause distortion of chest movement.

TECHNIQUE

The physiotherapist should explain to the patient the aims of the treatment and should point out the faults in his pattern of breathing; the use of a mirror may help. It may be helpful to demonstrate dia-phragmatic breathing to the patient before actually getting him to try it himself.

The patient should try to relax as much as possible first, then the physiotherapist should place her hands lightly on the upper abdomen overlapping the anterior costal margins. The patient should start by breathing out and at the same time relax the upper chest; if he is doing this correctly, the physiotherapist will feel the upper abdomen and anterior costal margins sink down and in. When the patient is ready to breathe in, he should be told to 'try to get air in round his waist' and if he does this correctly, the upper abdomen will bulge forward slightly and the anterior costal margins will move up and out. Many patients make the mistake of trying to take too deep a breath in and will expand the apical areas; this will inhibit diaphrag-matic movement.

Some patients find it very difficult to learn diaphragmatic breathing and many reverse the abdominal movement at first. It is vital to remember that the expiratory phase is completely passive; any forcing and prolonging of expiration will tend to increase airways obstruction.

Once the patient has mastered the technique, he should put his own hands in the correct place and feel his respiratory movements. He should be instructed to practise several times a day on his own (see Fig. 5/11).

Some physiotherapists prefer to place a hand lower on the abdomen when teaching diaphragmatic breathing commencing with a breath in; when doing this care should be taken not to allow the

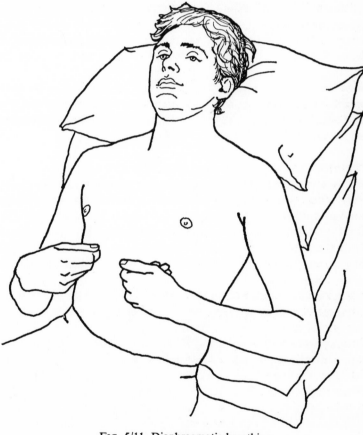

FIG. 5/11. Diaphragmatic breathing

patient to contract the abdominal wall on expiration as movements of the abdomen can occur that are not associated with breathing.

Use of Diaphragmatic Breathing During Attacks of Dyspnoea

If patients can be taught how to control their breathing during an attack of dyspnoea, this can be of great benefit to them.

The patient should be put into a relaxed position and encouraged to practise diaphragmatic breathing. The *rate* of respiration does not matter at this stage, it is how the patient breathes that is important. Every effort should be made to relax the upper chest and to get the patient to do quick gentle diaphragmatic breathing. As the patient gains control of his breathing he should be encouraged to slow down his respiratory rate.

There are five different positions that the patient can adopt when in distress.

1. HIGH SIDE LYING (Fig. 5/12A)
Five pillows are used to prop the patient up in bed, one of which is placed under the patient's side in order to wedge him up in bed and to keep his spine straight.

2. FORWARD LEAN SITTING (Fig. 5/12B and 12C)
The patient sits at a table resting the upper part of his chest against several pillows or the child sits or kneels with the upper chest supported on pillows.

3. RELAXED SITTING (Fig. 5/12D)
This is an unobtrusive, useful position that can be taken up easily.

4. FORWARD LEAN STANDING (Fig. 5/12E)
The patient can lean forward against an object of suitable height.

5. RELAXED STANDING (Fig. 5/12F)
The patient can lean back against a wall. The shoulders should be relaxed.

Localized Basal Expansion

This type of breathing is a useful method of trying to mobilize the

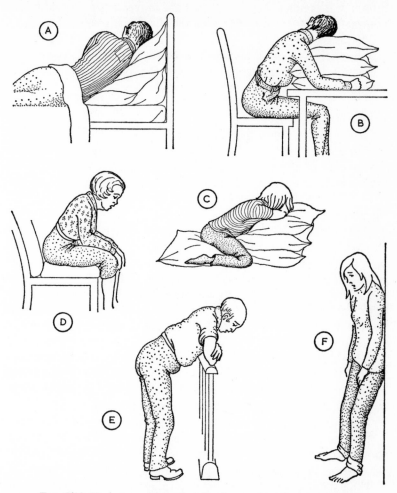

FIG. 5/12. Various positions that the dyspnoeic patient can adopt

lower chest and may make better use of the basal areas of the lungs. It should not be performed during attacks of dyspnoea as it requires extra effort. It can be taught bilaterally or unilaterally and is a 'trick' movement. It exaggerates the movement of ribs 8, 9 and 10, thus making better use of the outer fibres of the diaphragm. Some authorities state that it makes use of the 'bucket-handle' movement of the ribs, but there is a certain amount of controversy about this,

125

although it seems to be agreed that the movement is caused by the contraction of the outer fibres of the diaphragm when the central tendon is fixed.

When treating chest disease it is better to start off by teaching unilateral basal expansion, otherwise the patient is inclined to exaggerate the movement of the upper chest.

POSITION OF PATIENT

It is best to start with the patient in half-lying or sitting well supported so that he is unable to move his spine and thus simulate movements of the chest wall. Once the patient has mastered the correct technique he can sit upright and practise in front of a mirror.

TECHNIQUE

The physiotherapist should place the palm of her hand in the mid-axillary line at about the level of the eighth rib; her fingers should be well round the posterior aspect of the thorax. The patient should relax and breathe out feeling his lower ribs sinking down and in; at the end of expiration the physiotherapist should give firm pressure with her hand and instruct the patient to push with his ribs against her hand as he breathes in. Pressure should be released at the end of maximum inspiration.

If the aim of treatment is to re-expand lung tissue, the emphasis should be on holding the maximum inspiration for a short time before breathing out again, but if the patient has air trapping, the emphasis should be on relaxation during expiration.

The patient should be taught how to give pressure himself (see Fig. 5/13A) and some find it helpful to use a webbing band (see Fig. 5/13B). Some patients may have a stiff wrist or shoulder, in which case the back of the fingers or pressure by the opposite hand may be used.

The patient should be instructed to practise about 8 deep breaths at a time, then to rest before repeating 8 more, and so on. About 24 breaths at a time should be practised.

If the patient complains of dizziness, he is probably hyperventilating and should be told to pause longer between each breath.

Apical Expansion

This type of expansion is only necessary following certain types of thoracic surgery or when there is deformity of the chest wall or an

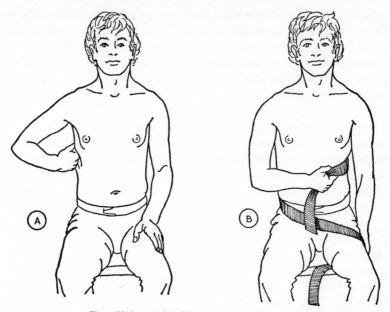

FIG. 5/13 A and B. The patient giving pressure

apical air pocket following spontaneous pneumothorax. It is not always necessary to teach apical expansion if there is disease in the upper lobe; a typical example of this is in cystic fibrosis when there is often involvement of the upper lobe but the patient is already over-expanding the upper chest.

POSITION OF THE PATIENT
The patient should be in a well-supported half-lying or sitting position. The physiotherapist should place her fingertips beneath the clavicle and encourage the patient to expand his chest upwards against her hand on inspiration. The patient can then be taught to give pressure himself with the opposite hand. This exercise should be taught unilaterally as it is only used for localized conditions.

If there is a persistent apical air pocket it is sometimes helpful to lie the patient flat on the unaffected side and tip the foot of the bed during breathing exercises.

Breathing Control on Stairs and Hills

Many patients with chest disease become very distressed when walking upstairs and up hills. If they can be taught to breathe in rhythm with their steps, this will often help them a great deal.

Each individual will vary, for example, some patients find it helpful to breathe out for two steps and in for one step, others prefer an even count. This does not matter so long as the patient breathes rhythmically with his steps. Many patients either hold their breath or breathe in an unco-ordinated manner on stairs and hills.

Once a suitable rhythm has been established, the patient should be encouraged to breathe with the diaphragm whilst walking. It should be impressed upon him that if he is half-way up a flight of stairs and is becoming distressed, it is better to stop and rest rather than trying to go on and having to sit down for 10 minutes afterwards to recover.

Other Types of Breathing Control

The physiotherapist can help breathless patients in other ways. Many complain of distress when they bend down—whenever possible they should kneel to do the task; if it is something like fastening shoe laces, they should breathe out as they bend forward.

INTERMITTENT POSITIVE PRESSURE BREATHING

Intermittent positive pressure breathing, commonly known as I.P.P.B., is a form of assisted breathing which can be a valuable adjunct to physiotherapy, particularly in the treatment of respiratory disease. It will provide more effective aeration of the alveoli and will aid the removal of retained secretions, and it is also a means of administering drugs directly to the airways.

Pressure-cycled machines with a patient-triggering mechanism are employed (see Intensive Care, page 78). The Bird and the Bennett ventilators are most commonly used for this type of treatment and various models are available. They are mainly driven by compressed gas (oxygen or air), but electrically powered ventilators are also obtainable, the latter being more suitable for use in the home.

In hospital, each machine should have several breathing head assemblies which will consist of tubing, nebulizer, exhalation valve and mouthpiece or mask; thus one ventilator can be used to treat several patients each day. There is no risk of cross-infection providing each patient has his own breathing head assembly, although precautions should be taken if a patient is infected with a resistant strain of bacteria. In this case the machine being used should not be moved to other patients, and should be sterilized with ethylene oxide gas when the patient concerned no longer needs I.P.P.B. The breathing head assemblies may be cold sterilized in a chlorinated disinfectant; Eusol, or a 1 in 10 solution of Milton, or Cidex, are commonly used.

Controls

The controls will vary slightly according to the make of ventilator, but basically are as follows:

1. THE INSPIRATORY PRESSURE LIMIT
This determines the maximum pressure generated by the ventilator. The pressure received by the patient is indicated by a gauge on the machine and should equal the setting; this will not be reached if there is any leak in the circuit, *e.g.* around the mouthpiece or mask, or if the patient breathes through his nose; under these circumstances the ventilator will not cycle into expiration. When patients exhale before the ventilator has reached the pre-set pressure, the needle on the gauge will swing round to a very high pressure.

2. THE AIR-MIX SELECTOR
When the ventilator is driven by oxygen this will entrain atmospheric air. The exact percentage will vary with the make of ventilator; some manufacturers state that the mixture is 40% oxygen and 60% atmospheric air, but this can vary a great deal.

3. THE EXPIRATORY TIMER
This will automatically cycle the ventilator but is not usually necessary for I.P.P.B.

4. THE SENSITIVITY CONTROL
This is used when the machine is to be 'patient-triggered' and can vary the amount of inspiratory effort needed to cycle the machine. It prevents the flow of gas during expiration until the generation of a small negative pressure by the patient causes the machine to cycle into inspiration. The sensitivity control can usually be adjusted so

that the slightest effort to breathe in on the part of the patient is sufficient to 'trigger' the machine into the inspiratory phase.

5. THE MANUAL CONTROL
Most ventilators have some means of manual control.

6. THE FLOW-RATE CONTROL
This mechanism is automatically incorporated in the Bennett and will vary with the inspiratory pressure settings. In the Bird, this control acts as an on-off switch and also controls the rate at which gas is delivered to the patient. At higher settings the flow-rate is increased so that the cycling pressure is reached sooner. This will reduce the tidal volume but as the overall respiratory rate per minute is increased the minute volume may be greater. To increase the tidal volume and allow deeper inspiration, the flow-rate control should be turned down. When the flow-rate is reduced and the machine is run off oxygen, the percentage of inspired oxygen will increase.

Preparation for Treatment

1. Fill the nebulizer with the prescribed solution. This solution should always be prescribed by the physician or surgeon in charge of the patient. Most nebulizers hold at least 5 ml of solution which will last about 15 minutes. Normal saline is frequently used but a bronchodilator may be ordered. For example, a 2·5 mg dose of salbutamol will consist of 0·5 ml of 0·5% salbutamol diluted with 4·5 ml normal saline. Glycerols are not usually suitable for use in I.P.P.B. nebulizers.

2. Connect breathing head assembly to the ventilator and connect the ventilator to the driving gas.

3. Set the controls of the ventilator. An average setting for the Bird Mark 7 is pressure 15, Flow-rate 7, Sensitivity 7, although these may have to be varied according to the requirements of individual patients.

4. Turn on the ventilator to check that the nebulizer is functioning correctly and that there are no leaks in the breathing head assembly.

Indications for Intermittent Positive Pressure Breathing

In some countries I.P.P.B. is used instead of physiotherapy, but it should only be used as an adjunct to physiotherapy when other measures have not been effective. Indications are as follows:

1. Sputum retention in medical and surgical conditions.
2. Hypercapnia, as in acute exacerbations of chronic bronchitis.
3. Severe bronchospasm as in status asthmaticus.
4. The re-education of paralysed respiratory muscles and as an aid to expectoration when this type of patient has a respiratory infection.

Treatment of the Patient

I.P.P.B. can be used to assist the removal of bronchial secretions, during postural drainage, but if bronchospasm is the dominant factor as in asthma, it is better to give a bronchodilator in the ventilator about 15 minutes before attempting to make the patient cough. These drugs may only be given 4-hourly.

Physiotherapists are often asked to treat patients in respiratory failure at the stage of impending coma. The patient is confused, drowsy and unable to cough effectively; in this situation the ventilator can be invaluable and intubation may often be avoided.

With this type of patient it is often necessary to use a mask and it is helpful to have another physiotherapist or a nurse to assist with the treatment. If possible the patient should be turned onto his side, one physiotherapist or the nurse should hold the mask over the patient's face, ensuring that there is an airtight fit and that the jaw is in the correct position, whilst the other physiotherapist vibrates the chest on expiration. The patient frequently becomes more rational and is able to cough effectively after about 10 minutes treatment, but it may be necessary to continue the procedure for longer. The patient should be watched for signs of drowsiness and if so, it should be reported to the doctor. If no results have been achieved after 15 minutes, naso-pharyngeal suction should be attempted. Treatment should be repeated for 15 to 30 minutes at 2, 3 or 4-hourly intervals, except during the night when the frequency of treatments can generally be reduced. As the patient's condition improves the number of treatments can be cut down and eventually discontinued.

I.P.P.B. can also be used in the re-education of paralysed respiratory muscles. Here the sensitivity should initially be set so that the effort required to initiate inspiration is minimal; by decreasing the sensitivity the patient will have to make more effort. In this way the

131

machine may be used to wean patients from non-triggered positive pressure devices or from tank respirators.

Maintenance of Equipment

It is advisable to have a supply of spare parts for the breathing head assembly as washers and springs will occasionally need to be replaced. It is also necessary to have the ventilators overhauled and cleaned every three months.

GENERAL EXERCISE

It is a well-known fact that many patients suffering from chronic pulmonary disease benefit from physical conditioning. It is also well known that asthma may be induced by means of exercise, although the exact mechanism still remains obscure. Bearing these factors in mind, physiotherapists should be prepared to change their approach to exercise in the treatment of patients with pulmonary diseases as more research is done in this field.

Children enjoy classes and for young patients with *cystic fibrosis* or *bronchiectasis*, an energetic class with plenty of running and jumping helps to loosen secretions before postural drainage. As these patients grow older, they prefer to take an active part in sport at school and they should be encouraged to do this as it is a boost to their morale to be able to compete with their contemporaries.

At one time most patients with *asthma* were encouraged to attend classes. These consisted of fairly vigorous general and posture exercises interspersed with breathing control. In view of the recent work on exercise-induced asthma, swimming is obviously the best type of exercise for asthmatics, but if circumstances are such that the only way of treating these patients is in a class, the following precautions should be taken.

1. The peak flow or $F.E.V._1$ should be measured before the class. Those patients with a particularly low reading should not take part in the class that day and should be treated individually.

2. The more vigorous exercises should not last for more than three minutes at a time and should be interspersed with breathing control.

Older patients with *chronic bronchitis* or *emphysema* do not do well in classes and should be treated individually. Although relaxed shoulder girdle and trunk movements may help to a certain extent, most benefit will be gained by a graduated exercise programme. Levison and Cherniack (1968) found that the respiratory muscles of these patients consumed 35% to 40% of the total oxygen uptake compared to 10% to 14% in normal individuals, therefore there was only 60% to 65% of the oxygen available for exercising non-respiratory muscles. After training in breathing control, many of these patients will be able to tolerate graduated exercise reasonably well, but patients who develop either premature ventricular contractions or marked cyanosis during exercise may need supplementary oxygen. The type of exercise given will vary according to the facilities available; some hospitals will exercise the patients by means of bicycles and treadmills, others by means of graduated walks and increasing the number of stairs climbed each day.

Each individual patient must be carefully assessed and exercised within his limitations. It is hoped that further research will reveal more about the effects of exercise in certain types of pulmonary disease and that physiotherapists will be able to apply these findings to their work.

REFERENCES

Anderson, S. D., Connolly, N. M. & Godfrey, S. (1971). 'Comparison of Bronchoconstriction induced by Cycling and Running.' *Thorax*, **26**, 396.

Campbell, E. J. M., Agostoni, E. & Newsom Davis, J. (1970). *The Respiratory Muscles—Mechanics and Neural Control*. Lloyd-Luke (Medical Books) Ltd., London.

Fitch, K. D. & Morton, A. R. (1971). 'Specificity of Exercise in Exercise-induced Asthma.' *British Medical Journal*, **4**, 577.

Gandevia, Bryan (1963). 'The Spirogram of Gross Expiratory Tracheo-bronchial Collapse in Emphysema.' *Quarterly Journal of Medicine*, New Series XXXII, No. 125, 23.

Gaskell, D. (1970). 'The Bird Mark 7 Ventilator.' *Physiotherapy*, **56**, 360.

Grant, R. (1970). 'The Physiological Basis of Increased Exercise Ability in Patients with Emphysema, after Breathing and Exercise Training.' *Physiotherapy*, **56**, 541.

Innocenti, D. M. (1966). 'Breathing Exercises in the Treatment of Emphysema.' *Physiotherapy*, **52**, 437.

Levison, H. & Cherniack, R. M. (1968). 'Ventilatory Cost of Exercise in C.O.P.D.' *Journal of Applied Physiology*, **25**, 21.

World Health Organization (1961). 'Chronic Cor Pulmonale.' *W.H.O. Tech. Rep. Ser.*, No. 213, 14.

BIBLIOGRAPHY

See end of Chapter 8.

CHAPTER 6

Pulmonary Infections

by D. V. GASKELL, M.C.S.P.

PNEUMONIA

The term pneumonia indicates an inflammation of the substance of the lungs.

The *classification* of pneumonia can be based on the anatomical distribution of the disease and on the nature of the infecting organism.

1. LOBAR PNEUMONIA

This is a pneumonic consolidation confined to one or more lobes of the lung. It is due to infections by specific organisms which are blood-borne, the main one being the virulent pneumococcus of which there are several different types. More rarely, it may be caused by *Staphylococcus aureus* or Friedlander's (*Klebsiella pneumoniae*) bacillus.

2. BRONCHOPNEUMONIA

This is a consolidation occurring in patches around infected peripheral bronchi. It may be confined to a small area or it may be widespread throughout the lung. It is often caused by inhaled airborne organisms such as streptococci, haemophilus influenzae and non-epidemic strains of pneumococci. In its early stages tuberculosis starts as a localized patch of bronchopneumonia, but widespread tuberculous bronchopneumonia may occur.

3. VIRAL PNEUMONIA

This may be complicated by secondary bacterial infection.

4. INHALATION PNEUMONIA

This may vary from a small area of consolidation to severe suppurative infection following inhalation of infected material.

5. PNEUMONIA SECONDARY TO DISEASE OF THE BRONCHI
This is often associated with bronchial carcinoma or bronchiectasis.

LOBAR PNEUMONIA

This is the classical type of pneumonia and may occur at any age. It is most frequently associated with infection by the pneumococcus.

The pathology of lobar pneumonia is briefly summarized as follows. The first stage of spreading inflammatory oedema proceeds to the second stage of red hepatization in which the affected lobe is firm, airless and red in colour, often with petechiae (minute haemorrhages) beneath the pleura. Bronchi in the affected lobe may also be plugged with fibrin. The alveolar capillaries are congested with blood and the alveoli are filled with red blood cells and fibrin. The third stage is that of grey hepatization when the lung shows a greyish-yellow appearance; prior to this the bronchial arteries are blocked proximal to the affected lobe but they appear to open up at this stage. The alveolar capillaries become less congested during the stage of grey hepatization and the pulmonary arteries may become thrombosed. The neutrophils phagocytose the pneumococci but apparently do not kill them. As resolution occurs the alveoli are invaded by macrophages which engulf both the leucocytes and their contained pneumococci.

The onset of the disease is often preceded by an upper respiratory tract infection. The patient rapidly becomes ill with an abrupt rise in temperature, with shivering and occasionally vomiting. At the same time pleuritic pain frequently develops over the affected lobe and the patient's respirations become rapid, shallow and sometimes grunting. There may be a dry painful cough at this stage but the patient will soon start to cough up 'rusty' sputum due to particles of altered blood from the areas of red hepatization. Cold sores (Herpes labialis) often develop at this stage.

The face will be flushed and possibly cyanosed. The respiration rate is raised and there will be diminished movement on the affected side with pain on deep inspiration. Within the first 24 to 48 hours signs of consolidation will appear, there will be dullness to percussion over the affected lobe and bronchial breathing will be present; there may be signs of pleural rub or even pleural effusion.

135

Pulmonary Infections

The diagnosis will be confirmed by an X-ray. In the days before antibiotics were available, the patient remained very ill for 5 to 10 days, then, if he survived, the temperature would subside rapidly by 'crisis' or more slowly by 'lysis'. Nowadays, this process is nearly always cut short by effective use of antibiotics, the patient's condition beginning to improve within 48 hours of starting treatment. As the signs of consolidation disappear, they will be replaced by coarse rales due to liquefaction of the inflammatory exudate. At this stage the sputum will become more purulent and the pleuritic pain less. It is possible for the condition to resolve without sputum production.

Treatment

The question of whether the patient should be treated in hospital will depend on the severity of disease and the care available at home. The general practitioner will be able to abort many attacks of lobar pneumonia by the prompt use of antibiotics in the early stages of the disease. If the patient requires admission to hospital, treatment consists of general management, control of pleuritic pain, antibiotics, the use of oxygen and appropriate physiotherapy.

Occasionally a patient may be first seen at a very advanced stage of the disease. This may be due to late referral or to an overwhelming infection. In this case the correct antibiotic is vital and the sputum should be examined immediately. Occasionally in pneumonia complicating severe influenza, the larynx and trachea may be blocked by sloughed mucous membrane and bronchoscopy followed by tracheostomy may be required.

As soon as the patient's temperature has subsided he should sit out of bed and his activities should be gradually increased. Younger patients will obviously recover more quickly than those over the age of 60.

Full recovery may be delayed by *complications* such as:

1. Delayed resolution. If resolution is delayed for more than 2 or 3 weeks, the possibility of an underlying condition such as carcinoma or bronchiectasis must be suspected and investigated. The sputum should also be examined for tuberculosis. Slow recovery should be anticipated in patients suffering from diabetes, cirrhosis of the liver, chronic alcoholism or nephritis.

2. Pleural effusions may occur but usually subside within a week or two of treatment.

136

3. *Empyema* may occasionally occur if the effusion becomes purulent.

4. *Cardiac failure*, possibly complicated by cardiac arrythmia, may occur in elderly patients.

5. Other complications include *pericarditis, endocarditis and meningitis.*

Physiotherapy

Many milder attacks of lobar pneumonia are treated in the home by the general practitioner. The physiotherapist usually only treats the severe cases that are admitted to hospital.

The aims of treatment are to assist in the removal of secretions and to regain expansion in the affected area.

Early in the disease, during the stage of red hepatization, the physiotherapist may not be able to help much and any vigorous treatment will only aggravate pleural pain.

Some physicians will not order treatment until the patient starts to expectorate but others prefer the physiotherapist to see the patient from the beginning.

If treatment is ordered in the early stage of the disease, gentle diaphragmatic breathing and localized basal expansion, holding the breath on full inspiration, should be started. The patient should be encouraged to cough but if the lung is still consolidated, this may not be productive in which case the physiotherapist should not drive the patient; intermittent positive pressure breathing (I.P.P.B.) may be helpful in aiding removal of secretions in severe cases.

Once the stage of grey hepatization starts, the patient will be able to expectorate. Postural drainage should be given for the affected area. If there is severe pleuritic pain, only gentle vibration should accompany it but percussion may be started as soon as the pain improves. Diaphragmatic breathing and localized basal expansion should be continued and treatment carried out two or three times a day.

As the X-ray improves and the sputum decreases, the treatment can be cut down. If the patient has not expectorated for two days, the physician should be consulted about the possibility of discontinuing postural drainage. Breathing exercises should be continued until discharge from hospital and older patients may need help with ambulation.

BRONCHOPNEUMONIA

Bronchopneumonia is very common, particularly in the aged. It is very often associated with chronic bronchitis and may also occur post-operatively, particularly in heavy smokers.

The initial symptoms are those of acute bronchitis, but the patient gradually becomes more ill and more breathless and cyanosis increases. It can be differentiated from bronchitis by the presence of patchy bronchial breathing and by the presence of patchy shadows on the X-ray.

The temperature, pulse and respiratory rate will be raised and there may be signs of carbon dioxide retention. The patient may sound 'bubbly' and have difficulty in getting rid of his secretions which will be purulent. There will usually be basal crepitations but the signs of consolidation will be minimal.

In patients with advanced chronic bronchitis, an attack of bronchopneumonia may precipitate cor pulmonale. Treatment will be similar to that of lobar pneumonia but particular care must be taken over the use of sedatives and oxygen. The principles of oxygen therapy will be the same as those in acute exacerbations of chronic bronchitis.

Physiotherapy

Unlike lobar pneumonia, patients with bronchopneumonia have secretions from the early stages of the disease and should have vigorous physiotherapy immediately. Many of these patients have underlying chest disease and will go into respiratory failure unless prompt action is taken.

Postural drainage with percussion and chest shaking should be given for the appropriate area. The patient may be dehydrated and if the secretions are very thick, steam inhalations or mist therapy may help to loosen tenacious sputum.

If the patient is drowsy and will not cough effectively, intermittent positive pressure breathing in conjunction with postural drainage is often helpful. If there is associated bronchospasm a bronchodilator may be ordered. If the patient will not cough despite these vigorous measures, it may be necessary to perform nasotracheal suction in order to clear excessive secretions. Occasionally some patients are very difficult to suck out via the nose and in this case it may be helpful to insert a Magill airway and suck out the pharynx.

To begin with, two-hourly treatment may be necessary and if the patient is verging on respiratory failure, it may be necessary to continue treatment during the night. As the patient improves, postural drainage will be cut down and gradually discontinued. Diaphragmatic breathing and localized basal expansion are taught and early ambulation encouraged.

VIRUS PNEUMONIA

Typical outbreaks of virus pneumonia may be seen in the armed forces or in general practice in the absence of superimposed bacterial infection. The patients are often not ill enough to require admission to hospital. The disease starts with the usual symptoms of general malaise followed by a cough which may be paroxysmal. If pain is present it is usually retrosternal rather than pleural. Physical signs in the chest may be scanty. X-ray may reveal an area of consolidation with a ground glass appearance and varying distribution.

Treatment

A virus pneumonia usually resolves within two weeks without specific treatment, although tetracycline sometimes seems to help. If the condition fails to improve, the diagnosis of carcinoma or pulmonary infarct should always be borne in mind.

Physiotherapy

Breathing exercises may be ordered for these patients if they are admitted to hospital. Postural drainage is only necessary if they have secretions present.

INHALATION PNEUMONIA

These bronchopneumonias are mainly caused by inhalation of food or juices from the upper gastro-intestinal tract. They are particularly liable to occur in infants and old people, those with bulbar neurological lesions, those under sedation and during or after anaesthesia or alcohol intoxication. They may also occur due to achalasia of the cardia, pharyngeal diverticulum, hiatus hernia and oesophageal strictures.

Clinically, inhaled vomit may give rise to haemorrhagic pneumonia with gross pulmonary oedema. These patients may be gravely ill and may even require intubation and artificial ventilation.

Smaller amounts of inhalation may occur in bulbar palsies and diseases of the oesophagus and the patient may present with recurrent cough and sputum. Once the cause of the pneumonia has been recognized its treatment may prevent further pneumonia.

Physiotherapy

Prompt treatment by means of postural drainage and possibly intermittent positive pressure breathing is vital.

LUNG ABSCESS

A lung abscess is a necrotic, suppurative, cavitated lesion mainly due to infection by pyogenic organisms. But it is also associated with tuberculosis, fungal infections, necrosis in malignant tumours and infected cysts.

Causes

Inhalation of infected material is a common cause. This material usually comes from the upper respiratory tract and may come from infected teeth, dental extraction or tonsillectomy. Foreign bodies or vomit may also be inhaled. The infected material is inhaled into a bronchopulmonary segment leading to a pneumonia which breaks down to form an abscess. The contents are coughed up leaving an abscess cavity usually infected with a mixed group of organisms. Lung abscess may also be secondary to bronchial carcinoma or other forms of obstruction.

An abscess may develop in the course of staphylococcal pneumonia, Friedlander's pneumonia or tuberculosis. Rare causes include actinomycosis, infected hydatid cyst and extension of amoebic abscess of the liver through the diaphragm.

The site of the abscess is influenced by gravity. If infected material is inhaled by an unconscious patient the abscess will occur in the most dependent part of his lung, *i.e.* if he is on his back the apical segments of the lower lobes or the posterior segment of his right upper lobe are frequent sites for abscess formation.

Signs and Symptoms

Symptoms frequently appear within three days of inhalation of infected material. Malaise and fever are accompanied by cough and pleuritic pain. At this stage the disease is often mistaken for pneumonia and antibiotics are started. In the absence of treatment the disease progresses with fever, pleurisy and possibly dyspnoea and cyanosis. This worsens over a period of about 10 days after which the patient characteristically coughs up a large amount of pus which may be foul-smelling and frequently contains blood. Other cases may be less obvious in their onset.

There will be dullness to percussion together with rales and sometimes bronchial breathing; a pleural rub may also be heard.

Chest X-rays will reveal the segment of lung involved. To begin with the affected segment will be opaque but when discharge of the abscess has occurred, a cavity will be seen containing a fluid level. The X-ray of a breaking-down peripheral carcinoma is characteristic: the walls of the cavity are thick and irregular.

Treatment

This will consist of antibiotics and accurate postural drainage. If the response to treatment is not satisfactory or drainage is not occurring freely, a bronchoscopy should be performed to exclude any obstruction such as a carcinoma. Very rarely resection of the area may be necessary.

Physiotherapy

This will consist of accurate postural drainage. The X-rays, particularly lateral views, must be studied carefully in order to establish the exact position of the abscess. If a fluid level is visible the patient is likely to have copious, foul-smelling sputum when drainage is instituted; in this case his condition will improve rapidly and the abscess will quickly reduce in size. Treatment should be carried out two or three times daily, until sputum is negligible and the X-ray shows healing of the abscess. Breathing exercises are not necessary as the aim of the treatment is removal of secretions from the abscess cavity.

Postural drainage will not always be immediately effective, in which case the orthodox postural drainage positions should be varied in case the abscess has caused distortion of the bronchi. Gentle vibration may assist drainage, but percussion should not be attempted as there is always the possibility of haemoptysis occurring. If postural drainage is still not effective after two or three days, the physician will probably consider a diagnostic bronchoscopy.

BRONCHIECTASIS

Bronchiectasis is a dilatation of the bronchi usually associated with obstruction and infection.

Causes

Bronchiectasis can be congenital but in most patients it is an acquired condition. It may follow inadequately treated pneumonia, particularly that associated with whooping cough (pertussis) or measles in which the mucus is thick and viscid causing obstruction and small areas of collapse. At this stage in the illness permanent bronchiectasis can be prevented if the obstructing plugs can be removed by vigorous physiotherapy.

Bronchiectasis may also develop when infection occurs distal to a bronchial obstruction caused by bronchial carcinoma, adenoma or external pressure from primary tuberculous glands. It may be associated with pulmonary infection which heals by fibrosis as in tuberculosis. It seems possible that bronchiectasis may follow bronchiolitis in infants and it commonly develops from the suppurating bronchiolitis in cystic fibrosis.

Mechanism and Changes

If a bronchus is obstructed air cannot reach the smaller airways and alveoli distal to the block. The air within them is gradually absorbed and all the smaller branches and alveoli collapse. The larger bronchi, which are held open by C-shaped cuffs of cartilage, remain patent. Should obstruction persist and infection supervene, certain changes follow because the products of inflammation are unable to escape along the airways. The alveoli undergo pneumonic consolidation which may lead to destruction of their walls and replacement by scar tissue. The smaller bronchi and bronchioles are obliterated, the in-flamed large bronchi lose their rigidity and elasticity and tend to dilate. It is thought that the dilatation is partly due to the damming back of secretions and partly because of shrinkage of the surrounding lung tissue caused by fibrosis.

The effects of these changes can be clearly seen in a bronchogram which will reveal varying degrees of dilatation of larger bronchi and failure to fill of smaller bronchi and bronchioles (see Fig. 6/1).

(a)   (b)   (c)

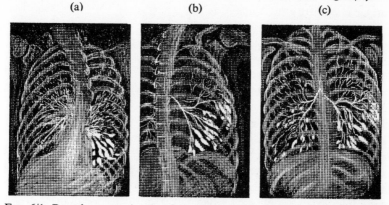

FIG. 6/1. Bronchograms showing bronchiectasis: (a) shows involvement of left lung; (b) shows involvement of middle and lower lobes; (c) shows involvement of both lungs

Signs and Symptoms

Cough and sputum are classical symptoms of bronchiectasis. The cough is often associated with change of position since this causes accumulated secretions to leave the cavities and come in contact with healthy bronchial mucous membrane and thus stimulate the cough reflex.

The sputum is usually purulent and in advanced cases several ounces may be coughed up in 24 hours.

Haemoptysis of varying severity may occur. Oddly enough the most severe haemoptysis is found in patients with relatively little previous history of cough and sputum. The middle lobe is the most common site of severe bleeding which may follow erosion of an artery by a 'broncholith'—a nodule of calcium derived from a lymph gland affected in a primary tuberculous complex. When haemoptysis is the only symptom the condition is sometimes known as a 'dry bron-chiectasis'.

On examination of the respiratory movements some flattening of the thoracic wall over the diseased lobe may be noticed and movement may be diminished in this area, which is a sign of fibrosis. Usually vital capacity is also decreased.

The general condition of the patient will vary considerably depending on the extent of the disease. Some patients look ill, have clubbing of the fingers, dyspnoea and copious quantities of sputum, while others are well apart from repeated chest infections following upper respiratory tract infection.

Complications

Repeated attacks of pneumonia are liable to occur either in the affected area or due to 'spill-over' of infected sputum into other areas of the lung. Cerebral abscess is a classical complication. Pleural effusion and empyema are relatively rare in previously diagnosed bronchiectasis, but underlying bronchiectasis is not uncommon in chronic empyema, presumably the original infected collapse giving rise to both conditions. Many patients have associated sinusitis and some physicians feel that this is the cause of the condition, infected material being inhaled into the lungs during sleep. Other physicians feel that the infection affects the respiratory tract as a whole.

Prognosis

If the material causing an obstruction is expectorated before changes actually occur then air will enter the collapsed area of lung and full restoration to normal should take place, but if the obstruction is not relieved early permanent damage occurs.

In the period before the use of antibiotics the prognosis of severe bronchiectasis was poor but with modern medical and surgical treatment, the prognosis has improved. Longterm survival will depend on the amount of lung destruction and the amount of generalized bronchitis. If the disease is very localized the patient may be cured by surgery. In the majority of patients symptoms may be reasonably well controlled, but not abolished, by means of antibiotics and postural drainage.

Most patients are able to lead a reasonably normal life apart from chronic cough and sputum, and more frequent respiratory infections than other people.

Treatment

The main object of treatment is to relieve the obstruction before permanent damage occurs. Thus efficient treatment of measles and whooping cough, removal of possible sources of infected material, and very careful prophylactic treatment to prevent post-operative lung collapse are all important.

Once bronchiectasis is established, prevention of accumulation of secretions will prevent further deterioration of the patient's general condition, subsequent complications and spread into other areas of the lung.

Conservative treatment consists of antibiotics and physiotherapy. If the disease is very localized or if there are repeated severe haemoptyses, surgery may be contemplated in order to resect the affected area.

Physiotherapy

In the conservative treatment this consists of clearing the cavities by accurate postural drainage, percussion and deep breathing exercises; training the patient in how to keep the cavities clear by postural drainage at home (see page 120); encouraging better use of all areas of the lung by breathing exercises (see Chapter 5, page 121); and encouraging exercise and sport in the younger patient.

If resection is to be undertaken, pre- and post-operative physiotherapy on the lines indicated in Chapter 10 is essential.

CYSTIC FIBROSIS

Cystic fibrosis is an hereditary disease affecting the exocrine glands. The main abnormalities are increased secretion of mucus and a high sodium chloride content of sweat. Most of the clinical abnormalities are related to obstruction by viscid mucus; the lungs, paranasal sinuses, pancreas and intestine are particularly affected. Bronchial obstruction by viscid mucus leading to secondary infection and lung damage is the commonest cause of death.

The disease is transmitted by a recessive gene and it has been calculated that 1 in 20 of the population may carry this.

145

Clinical Features

One of the earliest manifestations of the disease is acute intestinal obstruction at birth resulting from *meconium ileus*, which occurs in about 10% of cases. Others may present with symptoms suggesting *pancreatic insufficiency*, these include failure to thrive despite a good appetite, frequent large, foul-smelling stools and a protuberant abdomen. Many present with *respiratory symptoms* varying from recurrent cough to severe pneumonia. The cough is characteristically paroxysmal and violent. Following repeated infections, bronchiectasis will develop and there may be finger clubbing. Thick purulent sputum will be expectorated. There may be associated emphysema and cor pulmonale may develop during the course of a severe infection or in the terminal stages.

Diagnosis

Early diagnosis is of vital importance and any child or young adult with chronic or recurrent respiratory infection should be suspected of having cystic fibrosis, especially if relevant gastro-intestinal symptoms are present. The sodium chloride content of the sweat must be estimated; in children suffering from cystic fibrosis the concentrations of both sodium and chloride are over 70 mEq/litre in the sweat. This test is less reliable in adults.

Prognosis

At one time it was unusual for children with cystic fibrosis to survive over the age of 14. However in recent years early diagnosis and prophylactic treatment have considerably improved the prognosis with many patients surviving into their twenties and thirties.

Treatment

Many of these patients are treated at special centres where the staff have experience in the treatment of the disease and are able to instruct the parents in the care of the child.

Intestinal obstruction caused by meconium ileus will require surgical treatment but otherwise treatment will consist of maintaining nutrition, encouraging drainage of the respiratory tract and the control of pulmonary infection.

A high calorie and high protein diet with some restriction of fat and starch should be given with supplements of pancreatin and vitamins A, D and E. Additional salt and fluid should be given in feverish states or in hot weather, to replace the loss in the sweat.

Prevention and treatment of pulmonary complications by means of antibiotics and effective bronchial drainage are of vital importance. Mist therapy may be given in order to reduce the viscosity of the sputum. If wheezing is present a bronchodilator may be given. Emphasis should be placed on prophylactic treatment in the early stages of the disease. For patients with established lung damage, treatment should be guided by the clinical response.

Physiotherapy

Physiotherapy has a vital role to play in the treatment of cystic fibrosis. As soon as the diagnosis has been confirmed, a regime of postural drainage must be instituted and the patient and his relatives should be instructed in how to carry out postural drainage at home. This should be done once or twice daily for up to 30 minutes at a time depending on the amount of secretions present. If the X-ray shows that specific segments of the lung are involved, the appropriate postural drainage positions should be used. Otherwise the basal areas and mid-zones should be drained each day.

Patients with cystic fibrosis should be encouraged to take as much active exercise as possible; this will not only help to loosen secretions but will also boost their morale when they find they can compete in sports and games.

Breathing exercises should also be taught as some patients develop chest deformities. They should include diaphragmatic breathing and localized basal expansion. Apical expansion is not necessary.

During *acute exacerbations* physiotherapy must be stepped up. The patient may be admitted to hospital for intensive treatment and postural drainage may be given up to six times a day for 45 minutes at a time. It is often better to drain different areas of the lung at different sessions, *e.g.* the basal areas may be drained at one session and the mid-zones at the next session. If secretions are particularly tenacious, mist therapy should be given before or during treatment. If reversible airways obstruction is apparent, a bronchodilator given before postural drainage may be helpful.

In the terminal stages of the disease, treatment should be according to the patient's tolerance and it may not be possible to clear the chest completely each time. Treatments will be shorter and should not cause unnecessary distress to the patient.

Most physicians like patients with cystic fibrosis to visit the physiotherapy department when they come to the out-patient clinic; in this way the physiotherapist can check that the patient is carrying out his treatment correctly at home and can discuss any relevant problems with the patient and his relatives.

PULMONARY TUBERCULOSIS

Infection with the tubercle bacillus in an individual who has not previously experienced contact with the organism is called *primary tuberculosis*; re-infection after the primary lesion is called *post-primary tuberculosis. Miliary tuberculosis* is produced by acute diffuse dissemination of tubercle bacilli via the bloodstream.

In most countries in the western hemisphere, infection is almost entirely with the human bacillus, which is spread by droplet infection. In less economically developed countries, milk still serves as a vehicle for infection with the bovine organism causing primary abdominal tuberculosis.

People vary greatly in their susceptibility to the disease. Susceptibility may be inborn, but the disease is not hereditary. Resistance may be lowered by malnutrition, overwork and lack of sleep. The risks of infection are increased by proximity, either from overcrowded housing or by individual exposure, *e.g.* staff looking after patients with the disease.

Deaths from tuberculosis fell steadily in all civilized communities from the turn of the century, probably because of improved public health measures. Since the introduction of effective chemotherapy death rates have declined precipitously.

Investigations

The Mantoux test is used to determine the presence of antibodies to the tubercle bacillus. 0·1 ml of fluid containing extracts of dead bacilli (tuberculin) is injected in' radermally. This antigen reacts with any antibody present to produce a red indurated papule two to four days after the injection. A papule of 5 mm diameter is regarded as a positive result. Tuberculin is prepared in different strengths and a second injection with more concentrated tuberculin may reveal the presence of antibodies undetected by the weaker solution. Positive tuberculin reactions are found in patients who have been exposed to the bacillus at some stage in their lives. The reaction is more strongly positive during an infection. Negative reaction indicates that the patient has never been infected, although in overwhelming miliary tuberculosis negative reactions are also seen. Thus the Mantoux test is of limited value in diagnosis.

The most important investigations for pulmonary tuberculosis are sputum culture and chest X-ray. The latter may reveal shadows at the lung apex, enlarged hilar glands, or the widespread shadowing (mottling) of miliary tuberculosis. Smears of sputum are stained immediately and tubercle bacilli may be identified if they are present in large numbers. Sputum, laryngeal swabbings or aspirated gastric juice are cultured to identify the bacillus and determine its sensitivity to drugs; this process takes some weeks.

Occasionally enlarged neck or mediastinal glands are surgically removed for microscopic examination and mycobacterial culture.

Primary Tuberculosis

A small pneumonic lesion (Ghon focus) may present in any part of the lungs and the local lymph glands become enlarged. The radiographic appearance of a small shadow in the lung associated with hilar adenopathy is known as the primary complex. This is accompanied by a change in the Mantoux reaction to positive.

There is usually little upset in health and the natural tendency is to heal by fibrosis and calcification. In the past, primary tuberculosis was very common in young people and up to 1950 over 95% of the urban population had unknowingly healed such lesions before reaching adult life.

If the infection is severe, the child may appear to be vaguely unwell with reduced appetite, fretfulness and failure to gain weight normally. Cough is relatively unusual. Wheeze sometimes occurs and may be unilateral.

As tuberculosis is now less common, an increasing number of children reach adulthood without infection and protection should be given by means of vaccination by B.C.G. around the age of 13 if the Mantoux test is negative. (This is an attenuated strain of the tubercle bacillus, Bacille Calmette-Guerin.)

COMPLICATIONS

In young adults the lesion may spread throughout a lobe and occasionally cavitate. Primary tuberculous pleural effusions may occur.

In infants and young children, the enlarged hilar lymph nodes may cause compression of a bronchus and segmental collapse. This may lead to permanent bronchiectasis as in the middle lobe syndrome. An infected lymph node may also rupture through the wall of the bronchus and cause a widespread tuberculous bronchopneumonia.

TREATMENT

In any patient with a radiographically visible lesion, chemotherapy should be started and continued for a minimum of 18 months. The drugs most commonly used are isoniazid, streptomycin and para-aminosalicylic acid (P.A.S.). If the child is ill or febrile, bed rest is indicated. Providing chemotherapy is effectively administered, bed rest is otherwise unnecessary for the healing of the disease.

Postprimary Pulmonary Tuberculosis

The infection frequently occurs in the upper lobes or in the apical segments of the lower lobes. The early lesion is a small area of tuberculous bronchopneumonia which radiographically appears as a soft shadow of about 1 cm in diameter.

Spread will be by direct infection of adjacent lung tissue. Later caseation occurs and the necrotic centre of the lesion is discharged into a bronchus. This produces a cavity in the lung and the patient will have a cough with sputum. The infected sputum may cause bronchogenic spread of the lesion to other parts of either lung. Haemoptysis may occur if there is erosion of blood vessels.

The rate of progress of the disease is variable, depending on the extent and severity of the original infection and on the patient's resistance. Occasionally it progresses rapidly, but more often it takes some years to develop into widespread tuberculosis. The disease may become arrested at any stage, either permanently or temporarily, due to spontaneous healing by resolution, fibrosis and calcification or as a result of treatment.

As opposed to the acute tuberculosis described above, a state of chronic fibro-caseous or fibroid tuberculosis may develop with gross fibrous contraction of the upper lobe and compensatory emphysema of the lower lobes. Respiratory reserve will be diminished and dyspnoea and cyanosis may develop.

CLINICAL FEATURES

Many patients with early pulmonary tuberculosis may be symptom-free. The disease is often well advanced by the time symptoms have developed. Classically they are general malaise, cough with mucoid sputum, low-grade fever, anorexia, tiredness, progressive weight loss and night sweats.

SIGNS

There are no abnormal physical signs in an early lesion. If there is considerable lung involvement there is usually a small area of persistent fine rales at one or other apex. With extensive disease there will be impairment to percussion, widespread rales and occasionally areas of bronchial breathing. Fibrosis of an upper lobe leads to shift of the trachea towards the lesion with flattening and diminished movement of the upper chest. Signs of fluid will be present if there is an associated pleural effusion or empyema.

TREATMENT

The physician has to decide whether the clinical and radiological findings justify treatment and if so, whether the patient should be admitted to hospital. He also has to decide on which drugs to use.

In the past, many patients were admitted to sanatoria for prolonged bed rest, but nowadays only patients who are ill or who have extensive disease are admitted to hospital, and also those whose sputum is positive on direct smear or those who, because of the radiological extent of their disease, are likely to prove an infectious risk. Most patients remain in hospital for three months until three successive sputum specimens have been found negative on culture. (Sputa are only reported negative after being kept for two months.)

The standard drugs used are isoniazid, streptomycin and para-aminosalicylic acid (P.A.S.). They will be given for at least 18 months; many patients will continue them for about two years and a few patients with advanced disease may continue for longer. *No drug should be given alone or intermittently.* Failure to take combinations of the drugs without missing any doses may result in the emergence of drug-resistant strains of tubercle bacilli. If this unfortunate state of affairs should occur, certain reserve drugs are available, but most of them have side-effects and are expensive; the patient will require very careful handling in order to get him to persist with treatment.

Occasionally resection may be considered if the patient's organisms are resistant to two or more of the standard drugs, if the disease is localized and the respiratory function good, or if a cavity with thick fibrous walls does not heal.

Miliary Tuberculosis

This is caused by diffuse dissemination of the tubercle bacilli via the bloodstream. As the disease is frequently fatal without adequate treatment but recovery is the rule if proper chemotherapy is given, correct diagnosis is of vital importance.

CLINICAL FEATURES
The onset is usually insidious with general malaise, pyrexia, loss of weight and sweats. Evidence of miliary spread is not obvious early in the disease, but later a cough will develop. In some cases the patient presents with tuberculous meningitis.

Chest signs are either absent or confined to scattered fine rales. The spleen may be palpable and the retina may show choroidal tubercles. The chest X-ray shows the typical fine mottling of miliary tubercles throughout the lungs.

TREATMENT
Will be along the lines as for primary tuberculosis.

Tuberculoma

A tuberculoma is a cavity with thick walls, full of inspissated material. It shows on the chest X-ray as a rounded opacity with clear-cut edges and may contain areas of calcification. As it is often very difficult to differentiate between a tuberculoma and a carcinoma, some patients may undergo surgery and only then is the diagnosis definitely established. These patients will be given the usual anti-tuberculous drug therapy.

Physiotherapy for Tuberculosis

Although physiotherapy is not indicated in the treatment of tuberculosis, it may be used in the treatment of associated complications and in pre- and post-operative treatment (see Chapter 10, page 205).

Occasionally patients may be diagnosed as having bronchopneumonia and physiotherapy will have started before the diagnosis of tuberculosis has been made. In this case physiotherapy should be discontinued once the diagnosis has been confirmed.

Physiotherapy may be ordered for the following conditions:—

Tuberculous Pleural Effusion or Empyema

Once medical treatment has been instituted by means of aspiration and anti-tuberculous drugs, there is no risk of physiotherapy causing spread of the disease and it has an important part to play in the prevention of chest deformity and the loss of respiratory function due to calcification and thickening of the pleura.

The patient should be given localized expansion exercises to all areas of the affected side of the chest, attention being paid to the apical area even though the effusion is usually in the posterior basal area.

Belt exercises are often helpful and the patient should be encouraged to practise several times a day.

If severe chest deformity occurs, the patient should lie on his unaffected side with two pillows under his thorax in order to open out the ribs on his affected side. He should take up this position for half an hour at a time at least four times a day and should be encouraged to practise intermittent expansion exercises whilst in this position.

Treatment should be continued until chest expansion is equal and the X-ray has improved.

Middle Lobe Syndrome

Physiotherapy is often ordered for children with a collapsed middle lobe due to pressure from primary tuberculous glands. Although results are frequently disappointing it is worth persevering with postural drainage, vibrations and breathing exercises as some children obtain benefit from it. The physiotherapist should frequently review the situation with the physician, particularly if no improvement has been obtained after about two weeks' treatment.

Tuberculous Bronchiectasis

Some patients have associated bronchiectasis and will require postural drainage for the affected area. It is wiser not to percuss the chest owing to the danger of haemoptysis and the physiotherapist should always stand behind the patient when he is coughing. Treatment should be given two or three times daily according to the amount of sputum.

Associated Asthma or Bronchitis

Physiotherapy may be ordered for asthmatic or bronchitic patients with tuberculosis, when the treatment will be on the same lines as that for ordinary asthma or bronchitis (see Chapter 7), except that intermittent positive pressure breathing should not be given if there are any signs of cavitation, as this would be detrimental to healing.

CHAPTER 7

Chronic Bronchitis, Emphysema and Asthma

by D. V. GASKELL, M.C.S.P.

CHRONIC BRONCHITIS

The following definition of chronic bronchitis was approved by a committee of the World Health Organization in 1961:

'Chronic bronchitis is a chronic or recurrent increase above the normal in the volume of mucous secretion sufficient to cause expectoration, when this is not due to localized bronchopulmonary disease. The words "chronic" or "recurrent" may be further defined as "present on most days during at least three months of each of two successive years".'

Causes

Cigarette smoking and atmospheric pollution are two factors that are the main cause of hypersecretion. Infection is probably most important in causing irreversible lung damage.

Changes

The fundamental pathological change is hypertrophy of the mucous glands in the walls of the bronchi and an increase of goblet cells in the epithelial lining of the bronchial tree. This causes an excessive production of mucus (see Fig. 7/1).

At the same time, the cilia are unable to discharge the excessive mucus and have no more than a churning action upon it. These factors add to the obstruction of the airways.

155

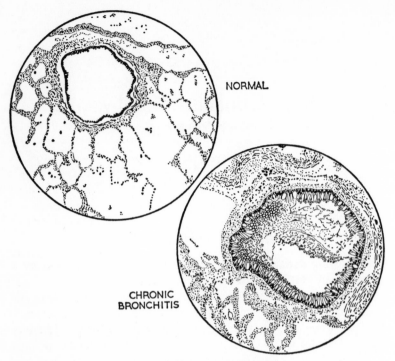

NORMAL

CHRONIC
BRONCHITIS

FIG. 7/1. Diagram of bronchioles

The excessive mucus in the bronchi predisposes the patient to infection. Where this is limited to the large- and medium-sized bronchi, serious impairment of respiratory function is unlikely. If it extends to the periphery of the lung and causes acute bronchiolitis and bronchopneumonia, the lobules may fail to resolve the exudate and may be replaced by fibrosis and contractures. Thus repeated infections over the years progressively reduce the number of patent airways and the area of effective alveolar surface.

The contraction of several lobules causes adjacent healthy lobules to expand and the individual alveoli become larger since many of them have previously been involved in acute inflammation and their weakened walls tend to rupture. In addition the scarred and distorted bronchioles often become kinked on expiration and cause air-trapping. These mechanisms lead to the development of secondary emphysema.

Signs and Symptoms

Characteristic symptoms are cough, sputum, wheeze and dyspnoea. The patient may complain of increasing disability following a recent infection, but on close questioning he will usually reveal that he has had a smokers' cough for many years.

As the disease develops the cough gradually becomes more continuous and frequently a bout of coughing occurs when the patient lies down. Upper respiratory tract infections tend to 'go down to the chest', when the sputum becomes purulent and increases in volume. To begin with the exacerbations may be fairly mild but later they cause increasing wheeze and dyspnoea and last for longer periods.

At a relatively early stage the patient's cough is exacerbated by fog and symptoms become worse during foggy weather.

There is considerable variation in individuals as to whether cough, sputum, wheeze or dyspnoea are the predominant symptoms.

Some patients may have a certain amount of reversible airways obstruction whilst in others it may be mainly irreversible due to a predominant emphysematous factor.

In the early stages of the disease the patient's general condition may be fairly good but in the later stages he may develop cor pulmonale (see page 110) and may appear blue and bloated. If the chronic bronchitic patient develops bronchopneumonia he may go into acute hypercapnic respiratory failure.

Clubbing of the fingers is unusual but may be seen if polycythaemia is present or it may be due to additional complicating factors such as bronchial neoplasm or bronchiectasis.

In the later stages of the disease the chest is often barrel-shaped with kyphosis, increased anteroposterior diameter, horizontal ribs, prominent sternal angle and wide subcostal angle. It is seldom that this appearance can be reversed once it is established.

Movement of the chest wall is restricted and may be confined to the upper thorax. The patient may have to use the accessory muscles of respiration. In the advanced stages of the disease, if there is a marked emphysematous factor, there may be paradoxical movement of the lower part of the chest wall. (The lower costal margin is pulled inwards on inspiration due to the pull of the low, flattened diaphragm.)

On auscultation rhonchi are widespread particularly at the bases
157

of the lungs. In milder cases they may only be present on forced expiration. If emphysema is present the breath sounds will be diminished.

Treatment

In the early stages of the disease, prophylactic treatment is extremely important. Once chronic bronchitis is established there is no possibility of a permanent cure and the most that can be done is to try to prevent further damage and alleviate the patient's symptoms.

Sources of bronchial irritation should be reduced to a minimum and the patient must be persuaded to give up smoking. It may be advisable for him to stay indoors during foggy weather.

Antibiotics will be ordered during acute exacerbations and the physician will impress upon the patient the importance of starting these at the very first sign of an upper respiratory tract infection. Some patients may be put on to longterm antibiotics, bronchodilator drugs and occasionally corticosteroids. Diuretics may be ordered for patients in cardiac failure (see cor pulmonale, page 112).

In acute exacerbations controlled oxygen therapy is of vital importance, particularly in those patients with a permanently raised PCO_2 (see respiratory failure, page 110).

Physiotherapy

Physiotherapy is of benefit in all stages of the disease.

In the *early stages* of chronic bronchitis the patient should be given postural drainage for the basal areas of the lungs. As many of these patients are older, this is more comfortably done in alternate side lying with the foot of the bed raised 12–18 inches (30–45 cm) from the floor. In hospital this should be done at least twice a day for up to 30 minutes at a time; vibrations and shaking on expiration will often help in removal of secretions. It is important for the physiotherapist to teach the patient how to drain his chest at home and if the bed cannot be tipped, a comfortable drainage position should be devised; he should be encouraged to carry out postural drainage morning and evening until his chest seems clear (this may take about 10 minutes on each side). It is important to fit in this regime with the patient's life and he is far more likely to carry out postural drainage regularly if it is only for a fairly short period at a time.

Breathing control should be taught in the early stages of the disease in the hopes that chest deformity will be prevented. Many of these patients will have poor basal expansion. The patient should be taught diaphragmatic breathing in all the relaxed positions, also localized basal expansion. If an exercise regime is to be started, many patients are able to improve their exercise tolerance quite considerably at this stage.

In the *later stages* of the disease, treatment will have to be modified to a certain extent. Most patients with chronic bronchitis will still tolerate postural drainage although there may be extensive lung damage. Many of these patients benefit from I.P.P.B. given in conjunction with postural drainage. A bronchodilator may be used in the nebulizer as there is often a degree of reversible airways obstruction and the secretions are more easily mobilized and expectorated due to the more effective aeration of the lungs by the ventilator. Vibrations and shaking should be given on expiration. Treatment should be given two or three times daily. At this stage in the disease the patient will have developed faulty breathing habits and may well have the typical barrel-shaped chest. Although it may be impossible to reverse the chest deformity, the pattern of breathing may be altered by means of breathing control and the patient can be taught what to do when in distress. Controlled breathing on stairs and hills is important. If an exercise regime is started it should be modified according to the patient's tolerance.

During *acute exacerbations* the chronic bronchitic may go into hypercapnic respiratory failure and prompt treatment will be required. If the secretions can be removed and effective alveolar ventilation restored, the patient's condition will improve. Many of these patients are drowsy and unresponsive and it is helpful to use I.P.P.B. with a mask instead of a mouthpiece. The patient should be turned onto his side and the foot of the bed elevated. If he has severe secondary emphysema he may not tolerate being tipped and should just be rolled onto his side. Help will be required to hold the mask over the patient's face and it may be necessary to hand-trigger the I.P.P.B. machine.

Once effective ventilation has been established, shaking and vibrations should be given on the expiratory phase and often the patient will start to cough and expectorate spontaneously and his colour will improve. If there has been no response after 10 to 15 minutes, nasotracheal suction should be considered. Care must be taken not to overtire the patient and controlled oxygen should be given whenever the I.P.P.B. mask has been removed. Treatment should be carried out for about 20 minutes at two-hourly intervals for the first 48 hours. If a bronchodilator is being given, this should be used for alternate treatments at four-hourly intervals.

The patient should be carefully observed for any signs of increased drowsiness after treatment and if so, the matter must be reported to the physician as it may be necessary to run the I.P.P.B. machine off air with controlled oxygen added.

During the night, it may be possible to cut down the number of treatments between 10 p.m. and 6 a.m., but it is usually necessary for the nursing staff to rouse the patient to give him I.P.P.B. and encourage him to cough at least once during this period. After 48 hours many patients will show marked improvement and the number of treatments may be cut down. If the patient does not improve the physician will have to decide whether to intubate and ventilate him, but many physicians are reluctant to take this step when patients have severe chronic bronchitis. If the patient is intubated, treatment will be as described in Chapters 3 and 4.

EMPHYSEMA

'Emphysema is a condition of the lung characterized by increase beyond the normal in the size of airspaces distal to the terminal bronchiolus, *i.e.* the acinus' (Reid, 1967).

There are several pathological classifications of emphysema. The two main types are:

Panacinar emphysema when there is dilatation or destruction of the acinus. This has been graded according to the size of the holes.

Grade I —holes up to 1 mm in diameter

Grade II —holes up to 1–3 mm in diameter

Grade III—holes up to 3–5 mm in diameter

Grade IV—holes over 5 mm in diameter

Patients who die from primary or idiopathic emphysema are found to have panacinar emphysema of at least Grade III severity throughout most of the lungs.

Centriacinar or centrilobular emphysema when the dilatation is more proximal and affects the alveoli arising from the respiratory bronchioli.

160

Causes

Emphysema commonly occurs in association with obstructive airways disease (see page 108) and is also related to occupational lung disease (see page 169). This is known as secondary emphysema.

More rarely it develops as a primary disease without any previous history of chest disease. It seems possible that in some patients a genetic factor might be responsible for the development of primary emphysema not related to chest disease or smoking. Eriksson has described three members of a family developing emphysema at an early age, all of whom had dysproteinaemia with a marked reduction of a_1-antitrypsin (Eriksson, 1964).

Signs and Symptoms

Lung function tests will show a low F.E.V.$_1$ which does not improve following the administration of a bronchodilator, thus demonstrating irreversible airways obstruction. The residual volume will be increased and the pressure volume loop will show an abrupt swing to a positive intrathoracic pressure on expiration. These are both indications of air trapping.

The X-ray will show a low flat diaphragm (below sixth rib anteriorly) and a large retrosternal translucent area, due to excess air in the lungs. Bullae may be visible. Cardiovascular changes such as a narrow vertical heart (less than 11·5 cm), prominence of the pulmonary trunk, large hilar vessels and small lung vessels will be seen.

Owing to the loss of elasticity in the lung, the patient finds it difficult to breathe out, but paradoxically, the more effort he makes to breathe out the more distressed he becomes. This is because forced and prolonged expiration will cause earlier shut-down of diseased airways and consequent air trapping. The work of breathing will also be increased; some patients may have learnt the trick of 'pursed lip' expiration, which causes a certain amount of back-pressure and may prevent shut-down of the airways.

Many emphysematous patients are breathless at rest and have been described as 'pink puffers' because cyanosis is not usually noticeable as in the chronic bronchitic or 'blue bloater'. By major effort, the emphysematous patient is able to ventilate sufficient alveoli to keep

161

his blood gases normal, so that he appears pink. The absence of hypoxaemia tends to preserve a normal pulmonary artery pressure and spares him from cardiac failure.

On examination the thorax may appear over-inflated, basal expansion is diminished and the chest elevated by the accessory muscles of respiration; there may even be paradoxical movement of the lower ribs due to the pull of the flattened diaphragm, the whole pattern of breathing appears unco-ordinated and every breath out is an effort. In some patients it will be noticed that on expiration the jugular veins fill and the inward movement of the abdomen on expiration is interrupted by a 'flick' or 'bounce' as the outward flow of air is suddenly checked by the increase in obstruction.

Treatment

This will be mainly palliative in the prevention and treatment of infection. The patient should be taught to breathe with the minimum amount of effort and to make the best use he can of his remaining healthy lung tissue by means of physiotherapy.

Occasionally surgical treatment may be considered if a patient has a large bulla compressing areas of healthy lung tissue. The ultimate success of plication or resection of large bullae will depend on the severity and extent of disease in the remaining lung tissue.

Physiotherapy

The aims of treatment are to teach the patient to breathe with the minimum amount of effort and to try to establish a co-ordinated pattern of breathing. Aid in removal of secretions may be necessary.

The patient must first be taught to control his breathing. A simple explanation of the mechanics of breathing should be given and the faults in his breathing pattern should be pointed out to the patient. He should be placed in a comfortable, well-supported half-lying or sitting position and encouraged to relax his upper chest and shoulders. Gentle, controlled diaphragmatic breathing should then be taught with emphasis on completely relaxed expiration (Gandevia, 1963). The rate of breathing should not be slowed down as the patient would then tend to lose control and revert to an unco-ordinated pattern. If abdominal 'bounce' is noticed the patient should be encouraged to shorten his expiratory phase and breathe in a little sooner (Innocenti, 1966). When the patient has gained a certain amount of control he should be shown the various relaxed positions to adopt when in distress. Many patients suffering from orthopnoea find it more comfortable to sleep in the high side-lying position.

The next progression will be to teach the patient controlled breathing with walking and how to breathe on climbing the stairs. Certain patients with very severe emphysema may be unable to walk without oxygen and may be supplied with a portable oxygen cylinder. This type of very disabled patient may find it easier to walk with a high walking frame.

If the patient has excess secretions he must be taught how to cough effectively and modified postural drainage may be necessary. Many patients with emphysema become very distressed by conventional postural drainage positions. Some patients will tolerate lying flat without the bed tipped, whilst others will only be able to lie on their side propped up by several pillows. Shaking on expiration should be given in a suitable position and effective coughing encouraged. Many emphysematous patients cough ineffectively due to shut-down of the airways and have distressing paroxysms of coughing. They should be told to breathe in after every two or three coughs and in this way will avoid shut-down of the airways.

It may also be helpful to use I.P.P.B. in order to aid expectoration. It is worth trying this with a bronchodilator at first and then measuring the F.E.V.$_1$ before and after I.P.P.B. to see if there is any degree of reversibility present. If there is no response to the bronchodilator, saline only should be used in the nebulizer.

Having taught the patient breathing control and aided expectoration, the next aim of physiotherapy will be to attempt a certain amount of lateral basal expansion, thereby trying to produce a more normal synchronized movement of the thoracic cage. Some physiotherapists feel that this is unnecessary, but the writer has found it worthwhile to persevere with localized basal expansion although it will take some time to achieve. Miss A. E. T. Hooper of Melbourne gave a paper on this subject at the W.C.P.T. Congress in Australia and by means of cineradiography was able to demonstrate its effect (*Proceedings of the 5th W.C.P.T. International Congress*, 1967).

Some physiotherapists like to teach thoracic mobility and posture exercises to emphysematous patients, in which case the emphasis should be on relaxed movements in co-ordination with breathing. Any form of bending forward should be avoided as this will cause distress.

COMPENSATORY EMPHYSEMA

This may occur when a section of a lung contracts by fibrosis or collapse or is removed surgically. The rest of the lung expands to fill the space by over-inflation. This is known as compensatory emphysema and is not associated with any defect of function.

ASTHMA

The term 'asthma' refers to the condition of people with widespread narrowing of the airways which changes in its severity over short periods of time and which is not due to cardiac disease.

Three factors contribute to this bronchial obstruction: contracture of the bronchial muscle—true bronchospasm; oedema of the mucous membrane; plugging with viscid mucus.

Causes

It is generally accepted that the bronchi of patients suffering from asthma are 'hypersensitive'.

Cases of asthma have been divided into two main groups:

1. The extrinsic type, where there is a recognizable antigen, which is associated with a history of eczema, hay fever, urticaria etc. This type commonly occurs in children and young people with a family history of allergy. Reaction to external allergens can be demonstrated by skin tests, when a weal develops within 10 minutes of the intradermal injection of the allergen.

2. The intrinsic type where no antigen is recognized. This type usually occurs in people of 40 years or over who have no personal or family history of allergy. The disease is often associated with infections.

Although these two groups of asthma differ broadly in many respects, the division is a provisional one as allergic factors may in due course be demonstrated in the intrinsic group.

Though the precipitating factors are mainly allergy and infection, attacks may also be caused by vigorous exercise, atmospheric pollution and other non-specific factors.

Psychological factors must also be taken into account. Although it is doubtful whether psychological stress alone causes asthma there is little doubt that such distress exacerbates asthma in certain

164

patients. In these patients treatment is not likely to be satisfactory unless the situation is appreciated and the patient handled with sympathetic understanding, tact and firmness, and the difficulties eased as much as possible.

Symptoms

A classical attack of asthma is rapid in onset. The patient has difficulty in breathing out and this results in an audible wheeze. In very severe attacks the airways obstruction may become so severe that there is no longer an audible wheeze.

The frequency and duration of attacks vary considerably. If a very severe attack has continued for more than 24 hours, it is described as 'status asthmaticus' and the patient will require admission to hospital.

Cough frequently occurs during asthma attacks and may be distressing and non-productive in the early stages. Once the bronchospasm has been relieved, the patient is often able to cough up plugs of tenacious sputum and will experience considerable relief.

Many patients suffering from asthma develop a barrel-shaped chest due to over-inflation of the lungs, but even longstanding chest deformity may be reversed if the asthma is effectively dealt with. In the very young child with chronic asthma the sternum may be drawn inwards or there may be Harrison's sulcus. Older children tend to develop pigeon chest or the same type of barrel-chest as adults. They also frequently have poor posture. Fortunately even gross deformities may reverse to a surprising degree if the chronic asthma is relieved by treatment.

Investigations

Various investigations are carried out including tests for hypersensitivity and respiratory function tests. Examination of the blood and sputum for eosinophils is also helpful.

The most valuable respiratory function test is the forced expiratory volume in one second ($F.E.V._1$) and the forced vital capacity ($F.V.C.$). This can be measured at the bedside by means of a portable spirometer. A vitalograph or vitalor is often used. These are valuable means of assessing the patient's response to treatment.

Treatment

Treatment is by means of bronchodilators and sometimes cortico-steroids. An antibiotic may be prescribed if infection is present.

If a particular allergen has been identified, it is sometimes possible to avoid it or at least reduce exposure to it. In the case of house dust, it is particularly important to avoid accumulation of dust by making changes in the furnishing of the patient's bedroom and cleaning it very thoroughly. The mattress should be vacuum-cleaned every day. There is controversy over the value of desensitization, some allergists feeling that it is helpful in certain cases.

Disodium cromoglycate (Intal) is of use in inhibiting the patient's reaction to allergy and as a result of its prophylactic use, many asthmatic children are able to lead a much more normal life with very little loss of schooling.

Physiotherapy used in conjunction with medical treatment can be of great value in the treatment of asthma.

Physiotherapy

The physiotherapist will be asked to treat asthmatic patients whose condition will vary from severe status asthmaticus to those patients who have no symptoms at all at the time of treatment. In the former situation the aims of treatment will be to relieve bronchospasm and to assist in the removal of secretions, whereas in the latter situation the physiotherapist should teach the patient what to do when he has an asthma attack, assist in removal of any secretions present and try to teach a more efficient pattern of breathing. Obviously there will be many patients varying between these two extremes.

When a patient is admitted in *status asthmaticus* bronchodilators will be given in order to relieve bronchospasm and a very effective means of delivering these drugs is by I.P.P.B. If this equipment is available, the physiotherapist is often asked to treat the patient at this stage. The F.E.V.$_1$ or peak flow should be measured first and the patient should sit comfortably upright in bed and use the I.P.P.B. machine until the nebulizer is empty. Apart from encouraging the patient to breathe with his lower chest whilst using the machine the physiotherapist should not attempt other measures at this stage. If I.P.P.B. is not available, the physiotherapist should put the patient

166

in a high side-lying position and encourage gentle diaphragmatic breathing in the patient's own time. He will not be able to breathe slowly at this stage.

As the bronchodilator takes effect, the patient will be able to breathe more easily and may start to cough spontaneously. About 15 minutes after administration of the bronchodilator (either by I.P.P.B. or other means) the physiotherapist should position the patient in high side lying, gently vibrate the chest on expiration and encourage the patient to cough. Frequently he will expectorate tenacious sputum containing plugs and will experience rapid relief. The F.E.V.$_1$ or peak flow will demonstrate the improvement. However, some patients are unable to expectorate and if they persist in trying at this stage, the bronchospasm will become worse. Apart from making the patient comfortable and encouraging gentle diaphragmatic breathing, the physiotherapist should leave this type of patient until the drugs start to take effect. I.P.P.B. with a bronchodilator can be repeated at four-hourly intervals. As the patient's condition improves he will be able to lie flat and even be tipped in order to remove secretions.

Breathing control is of importance; it can be a great help to a patient during a mild attack of asthma. He should be told to get into a relaxed position and to try to breathe gently with his diaphragm, expiration should not be forced. In between attacks patients should practise this type of breathing and should also include basal expansion exercises. Many children with asthma develop quite severe chest deformities and faulty patterns of breathing; these deformities will disappear if the asthma is treated effectively. Breathing exercises will help to improve the faulty breathing habits.

Certain patients with asthma, particularly children, have secretions present at all times; in this situation, it is helpful if the patient carries out postural drainage each day in order to prevent accumulation of secretions. The physiotherapist should explain how to do this at home.

Many patients have exercise-induced asthma and research is being done in this field at the present time. If asthma patients are treated in classes, more vigorous exercises should not be done for more than three minutes at a time and should be interspersed with gentle breathing exercises. Asthma is less likely to be induced by swimming (Fitch & Morton, 1971) and this is a very effective form of exercise for these patients.

167

FUNGAL INFECTIONS OF THE LUNG

The main fungal infections of the lung (pulmonary mycoses) encountered in Britain are aspergillosis, candidiasis, actinomycosis and cryptococcosis.

Aspergillosis

This is the commonest fungal disease affecting the lungs. The Aspergillus thrives on decaying vegetation in warm, humid conditions and releases spores particularly through the winter months. *Aspergillus fumigatus* is the most common species responsible for aspergillosis in man. There are four different types.

ASYMPTOMATIC ASPERGILLOSIS

Many bronchitics have a few spores in their sputum. This is due to poor sputum clearance and the ubiquity of the spores. No special treatment is necessary.

ASPERGILLOMA

A solid ball of fungus (mycetoma) may grow in a pre-existing cavity. It commonly forms in an old tuberculous cavity and less frequently in cavities caused by lung abscess, pulmonary infarction etc. Radiographically a crescent of air may be seen over the ball of fungus which can be shown to change its position with changes of posture.

Some patients may be asymptomatic, others may have recurrent haemoptyses or repeated infections with thick purulent sputum.

Aspergilloma is often left untreated as there is always the risk of spread of infection during surgery and bronchopleural fistula may result. However, lobectomy may be undertaken if recurrent severe haemoptyses occur.

DISSEMINATED ASPERGILLOSIS

There may be spread of the disease into the lung and pleura with progressive destruction of the lung tissue; it may also spread to other organs. The patient is very ill and there is a poor prognosis. Treatment may be by amphotericin B given intravenously or pneumonectomy may occasionally be considered.

BRONCHIAL ASPERGILLOSIS WITH ALLERGIC MANIFESTATIONS

Some patients become allergic to the Aspergillus and about 2½ hours after exposure the bronchi and bronchioles become acutely inflamed, oedematous and haemorrhagic. Transient pulmonary infiltrates develop associated with fever, wheezing and eosinophilia. Bronchial casts, often brown in colour, may be coughed up from which *Aspergillus fumigatus* can be cultured. Obstruction of bronchi by mycelium can result in collapse of a segment or lobe or rarely, a lung.

Repeated attacks can cause bronchiectasis or the disease may spread into the alveoli and cause diffuse pulmonary fibrosis.

Treatment will be by means of various antifungal agents. Allergic bronchial aspergillosis may persist for years with episodes of wheeze, fever, eosinophilia and radiographic evidence of transient consolidation and collapse. Some patients will recover spontaneously, others develop severe chronic asthma and may need corticosteroids and bronchodilators in order to overcome symptoms.

PHYSIOTHERAPY

The aims of treatment will vary according to the patient's symptoms. Vigorous postural drainage will be necessary in order to remove bronchial casts, often an exhausting procedure for the patient and the physiotherapist. If wheezing is the main problem, treatment will be similar to that of asthma consisting of I.P.P.B., assisted coughing and breathing control. Treatment may be necessary three times a day.

Frequently the patient will be wheezy but will also have patchy areas of consolidation. I.P.P.B. with bronchodilators should be given first in order to relieve spasm, this should be followed by postural drainage for affected areas with fairly vigorous shaking of the chest; if the patient will not tolerate the correct postural drainage position it should be modified. Some patients will be having antifungal inhalations and if so, these should be given after physiotherapy when it is hoped the airways will be reasonably clear.

OCCUPATIONAL LUNG DISEASE

Damage to the lungs by dusts or fumes or noxious substances inhaled by workers in certain specific occupations is known as 'occupational lung disease'.

Coal Miners' Pneumoconiosis

This is a special type of pneumoconiosis due to the prolonged inhalation of coal dust, rather than rock dust which produces silicosis. It is most prevalent in the South Wales coalfields and there are two types.

1. Simple Pneumoconiosis. The X-ray shows diffuse reticulation at first. Later small scattered nodules up to 5 mm in diameter develop, often with surrounding emphysema. The disease is only progressive if the worker remains exposed to dust.

2. Progressive Massive Fibrosis. The X-ray shows large dense shadows mostly in the middle and upper zones with surrounding emphysema. At one time it was thought that this was due to a tuberculous infection superimposed on a simple pneumoconiosis, but it is now thought that fibrosis caused by an enhanced immune reaction occurs followed by the deposition of immune globulin in the pneumoconiotic lungs.

CLINICAL FEATURES

The diagnosis of pneumoconiosis should be suspected in a man who complains of increasing breathlessness on exertion and who has worked in the coal mines for several years. It is common for the patient to be a cigarette smoker and to have associated chronic bronchitis. If sputum is present it is usually mucoid but it will become purulent during infective exacerbations. It may become jet black when lesions cavitate. Once progressive massive fibrosis is established the disease is progressive even if the patient is no longer exposed to coal dust. In advanced cases, the patient becomes grossly disabled and death from cor pulmonale is usual. Pulmonary tuberculosis may develop as an added complication.

TREATMENT

There is no specific treatment for pneumoconiosis and the most important aspect of its management is prevention. This implies effective dust suppression, the early recognition of dust retention by means of routine radiography and when necessary, the provision of alternative employment in areas of low dust concentration to prevent progress of the disease.

170

PHYSIOTHERAPY

Physiotherapy will be similar to that used in the treatment of chronic bronchitis and emphysema (see pages 158 and 162). If the patient has an infection every effort should be made to assist in the removal of secretions. If there is extensive fibrosis, intermittent positive pressure breathing may be helpful in assisting the patient to cough. In the advanced stages of the disease, all that the physiotherapist can do is to try to teach the patient to breathe with the minimum amount of effort and to assist in effective coughing.

Silicosis

Silicosis is due to inhalation of fine particles of free silica $1–10\mu$ in diameter. It occurs in coal mines, in the granite and sandstone industries, in metal foundries, in various metal grinding processes and in the pottery industry.

CHANGES

The earliest is the development of fine fibrotic nodules around the particles of silica throughout the lungs. As the disease develops, these nodules increase in size and finally there are large areas of fibrosis. Tuberculosis may be a complication.

CLINICAL FEATURES

Symptoms do not usually develop until after several years of exposure to the dust. The chronic form of the disease usually presents with progressive dyspnoea on exertion, accompanied by unproductive cough and recurrent bouts of bronchitis. Occasional haemoptysis may occur. If tuberculosis supervenes there is deterioration in the general condition accompanied by increase in cough and sputum, pyrexia and loss of weight. Eventually the patient becomes very disabled and death occurs from bronchopneumonia, tuberculosis or cor pulmonale.

TREATMENT

There is no specific treatment and since silicosis continues to progress after exposure to the dust has ceased, it is vital to diagnose the disease early and remove the patient from further contact with the dust. All workers exposed to silica dust should have regular chest X-rays.

PHYSIOTHERAPY

The treatment will be as for chronic bronchitis and emphysema. The aims will be to help in removal of secretions by means of postural drainage and possibly intermittent positive pressure breathing and to teach the patient to breathe with the minimum amount of effort.

Asbestosis

This is a form of pneumoconiosis due to the inhalation of asbestos dust, causing a progressive fibrosis of the lungs, particularly the lower lobes. The main symptoms are cough and dyspnoea. Asbestos bodies can be found on microscopy of the sputum.

Preventative measures are similar to those used in silicosis.

Carcinoma of the bronchus is a common complication and malignant mesothelioma of the pleura also occurs.

Various other occupational diseases such as *Farmer's lung* will be encountered by physiotherapists treating chest disease. Details can be found in textbooks dealing with chest disease and physiotherapy will be directed towards assistance with expectoration and teaching the patient to breathe with the minimum amount of effort. I.P.P.B. may also be of help.

DIFFUSE FIBROSING ALVEOLITIS

This is alternatively known as diffuse interstitial lung disease, diffuse interstitial pulmonary fibrosis, Hamman-Rich syndrome.

It is a condition of unknown aetiology characterized by a diffuse inflammatory process beyond the terminal bronchiole. Essential features are cellular thickening of the alveolar walls showing a tendency to fibrosis and the presence of large mononuclear cells within the alveolar spaces.

Clinically the outstanding characteristic is progressive and un-remitting dyspnoea. Clubbing of the fingers is common. The disease is often fatal, in the subacute form originally described by Hamman and Rich this may be within six months, in the commonest chronic form within a few years.

The only effective treatment is with corticosteroid drugs. Other treatment is purely palliative. Oxygen is given in high concentrations,

172

as patients with fibrosing alveolitis do not retain carbon dioxide. In the later stages secondary infection may require treatment. Heart failure may be temporarily improved with diuretics and digitalis. Appropriate sedation should be given in the terminal stages.

PHYSIOTHERAPY

This will be purely palliative but may be of help during infections when I.P.P.B. and chest vibration may help in the removal of secretions. Positions for dyspnoea and breathing control during walking can also be taught to the patient in the early stages of the disease in the hope that they might help a little.

REFERENCES

Chronic bronchitis

Gaskell, D. V. (1966). 'Acute Exacerbations in Chronic Bronchitis.' *Physiotherapy*, **52**, 431.

World Health Organization (1961). 'Chronic Cor Pulmonale.' *W.H.O. Tech. Dep. Ser.*, No. 213, 14.

Emphysema

Eriksson, S. (1964). 'Pulmonary Emphysema and α_1-Antitrypsin Deficiency.' *Acta Med. Scand.*, **175**, 197.

Grant, R. (1970). 'The Physiological Basis of Increased Exercise Ability in Patients with Emphysema after Breathing and Exercise Training.' *Physiotherapy*, **56**, 541.

Hooper, A. E. T. (1967). 'Physical Therapy for an Emphysematous Patient.' *Proceedings of the Fifth W.C.P.T. International Congress*, pp. 119–33. Australian Physiotherapy Association, Melbourne.

Innocenti, D. M. (1966). 'Breathing Exercises in the Treatment of Emphysema.' *Physiotherapy*, **52**, 437.

Reid, Lynne (1967). *The Pathology of Emphysema*. Lloyd-Luke (Medical Books) Ltd., London.

Asthma

Fitch, D. & Morton, A. R. (1971). 'Specificity of Exercise in Exercise-induced Asthma.' *British Medical Journal*, **4**, 577.

BIBLIOGRAPHY

See end of Chapter 8.

CHAPTER 8

Pulmonary Embolism, Lung Tumours and Diseases of the Pleura

by D. V. GASKELL, M.C.S.P.

PULMONARY EMBOLISM

A pulmonary embolus most commonly arises from a deep vein thrombosis in the leg or pelvis. More rarely it may arise from an intracardiac thrombosis following atrial fibrillation or cardiac infarction.

CLINICAL FEATURES

It may present in different ways and it is important to distinguish between the signs of massive pulmonary embolism and pulmonary infarct.

Massive Pulmonary Embolism

This is defined as obstruction to more than 50% of the major pulmonary artery branches.

A large pulmonary embolism may cause sudden death; the classical description of an elderly, possibly obese patient around the tenth post-operative day calling for a bedpan and suddenly collapsing is well known. If the embolism is not immediately fatal, the patient becomes suddenly shocked and will complain of central chest pain, there will be distressing dyspnoea but not orthopnoea, and cyanosis and profuse sweating. The blood pressure will fall and the jugular venous pressure will rise; 60–85% of the cross-sectional area of the pulmonary arteries have to be occluded before the systemic blood pressure falls and only massive emboli can cause such acute ob-

174

structive pulmonary hypertension. There will be sinus tachycardia and a gallop rhythm. Pulmonary arteriography will confirm the diagnosis.

Pulmonary Infarction

Small emboli cause pulmonary infarction. There is frequently pleuritic pain and pleural effusion may develop; about 50% of patients have haemoptysis. Dyspnoea is variable and linked with the degree of pleuritic pain; there may be a varying degree of pyrexia present and tachycardia of over 100 per minute is found in the majority of cases. Symptoms are frequently slight and it is the most commonly overlooked serious respiratory lesion. It should be remembered that repeated small pulmonary emboli may seriously obstruct the pulmonary vascular bed and lead to pulmonary hypertension and right ventricular failure.

TREATMENT

Treatment is primarily prophylactic and is directed towards those patients at greatest risk—the old and obese, the patient with cardiac disease, the post-partum and post-operative patient. Acceleration of the venous return by means of exercise and early ambulation is important. Patients confined to bed should be examined frequently for the development of evidence of phlebothrombosis. If there is any suspicion of deep venous thrombosis, anticoagulant therapy should be started immediately unless there are strong contra-indications.

Massive pulmonary embolism requires urgent treatment and intravenous anticoagulants may prevent extension of the clot. Oxygen should be given freely and the usual measures for acute circulatory failure employed. Morphine or pethidine may be given for relief of pain and apprehension. Methods of treatment include the use of anticoagulants, fibrinolytic agents and emergency pulmonary embolectomy.

Treatment of pulmonary infarction will be by means of anticoagulant therapy, oxygen and bed rest. Morphine may be required for the associated pain.

PHYSIOTHERAPY

Treatment is mainly *prophylactic* and all patients at risk should be given active leg exercises and breathing exercises in order to assist the venous return. These patients should be encouraged to carry out active foot and leg movements at frequent intervals during the day.

If a pulmonary embolus should occur, physiotherapy should be discontinued until anticoagulant therapy has been established when treatment will be re-ordered by the physician or surgeon. At this stage some patients may cough up a certain amount of old blood and clot and chest movements may be limited due to pleuritic pain. Localized breathing over the affected area should be encouraged and it may be necessary to give postural drainage. Leg exercises should be continued until the patient is ambulant.

If a pulmonary embolectomy is performed, physiotherapy will be carried out on the same lines as for other patients undergoing cardio-pulmonary bypass (see Chapter 11, page 217).

TUMOURS OF THE LUNG

Carcinoma of the Bronchus

This is by far the commonest tumour of the lung and its incidence has greatly increased over the past thirty years. All the available evidence attributes the great rise in mortality from this disease to the smoking of tobacco, particularly cigarettes.

The majority of these tumours arise centrally either in, or proximal to, a segmental bronchus. A few are peripheral.

Histologically 56% are found to be squamous cell carcinomas, 37% are anaplastic (oat cell carcinomas), 6% adenocarcinoma and 1% alveolar cell carcinomas.

SYMPTOMS

A dry cough or a change in the nature of the cough is often an early symptom; haemoptysis may also occur. A persistent wheeze and dull, deep-seated pain are common symptoms.

As the growth increases in size it will cause progressive bronchial obstruction with mucopurulent sputum and eventual collapse of the segment.

In some patients the disease may be discovered by means of mass X-ray. Others may remain symptom-free until complications occur.

COMPLICATIONS

Inflammatory complications may present as pneumonia or lung

176

abscess. Any patient with a segmental pneumonia which fails to resolve, or recurs repeatedly in the same area, should be investigated for a bronchial carcinoma.

Pressure by the tumour may cause collapse of a lung segment or obstruct the superior vena cava.

Tumour cells may directly invade the pleura and cause pleural effusion or this may be the result of spread of inflammation. Again, the cells may infiltrate the pericardium or heart muscle causing atrial fibrillation or pericardial effusion.

Distal metastases may occur in any part of the body and endocrine and metabolic disorders occasionally occur.

Neurological complications are not uncommon. There may be involvement of the brachial plexus together with pain and weakness in the arm (Pancoast's tumour), or of sympathetic ganglia (producing Horner's syndrome). The recurrent laryngeal and phrenic nerves may be affected with resultant hoarseness and hiccough respectively.

Finger-clubbing with pulmonary pseudo-hypertrophic osteoarthropathy may sometimes be present. This causes pain and swelling in the joints, particularly the fingers, wrists and ankles. The X-ray will show typical subperiosteal reaction leading to new bone formation.

Any patient presenting with the above features should have a chest X-ray which may confirm the presence of bronchial carcinoma. The sputum should be examined for carcinoma cells which can be found in two cases out of three (Oswald *et al.*, 1971). If there is any doubt as to the diagnosis, bronchoscopy is carried out. It is always done if surgery is being contemplated in order to decide whether the tumour is operable.

TREATMENT

Apart from anaplastic (oat cell) carcinoma when radiotherapy may be the treatment of choice, the main hope of a cure lies in the surgical removal of the affected lobe or lung. Unfortunately many patients are not suitable for this type of treatment either because of the extent of the growth or because of poor respiratory function.

Radical radiotherapy may be considered but not all patients are suitable for this. If the disease is too advanced malaise produced by irradiation sickness may outweigh the benefit gained.

Palliative radiotherapy is more commonly used, in order to relieve symptoms and make the patient more comfortable, particularly for those with obstruction of the superior vena cava, pain, haemoptysis, distressing cough or obstruction of a large bronchus.

Cytotoxic drugs may be used in the treatment of malignant pleural effusion and antibiotics may be used for secondary infection.

In many cases only symptomatic measures are possible and with each individual the physician will have to consider carefully what he will tell the patient and his relatives. All possible measures should be taken to relieve physical and mental suffering.

PHYSIOTHERAPY

Physiotherapy is most often required for the pre-operative or pre-bronchoscopy preparation of the patient and in the post-operative treatment and is carried out on the lines indicated in Chapter 10.

If the patient is being treated by means of radiotherapy and if there is infection beyond the bronchial obstruction, as the tumour reduces in size and the obstruction is relieved, the patient will start to expectorate purulent sputum. This can be considerably facilitated by means of postural drainage. Gentle vibrations may be given but it is wiser not to give percussion and vigorous shaking in view of the possibility of haemoptysis or the presence of metastases in the spine or ribs.

A physiotherapist may be asked to help patients in the terminal stages of the disease if they are troubled by excessive secretions and if they are having difficulty in expectoration. It may be possible to help in the removal of secretions by means of postural drainage and gentle vibrations. Very occasionally nasotracheal suction may be contemplated, but this should only be done if the patient is alert and in extreme distress. The writer feels that this procedure should not be carried out in comatose patients in the terminal stages of the disease.

Some patients may develop pulmonary fibrosis as a result of radiotherapy. They will be short of breath and it may be helpful to teach them controlled breathing, particularly when walking (see Chapter 5, page 127).

Adenoma of the Bronchus

This is a benign tumour which rarely undergoes malignant change. It is less common than carcinoma of the bronchus and may present as haemoptysis or as bronchial obstruction with infection. Diagnosis is confirmed by bronchoscopy. The tumour is surgically removed.

Hamartoma

This is a benign tumour of the lung and it is composed of a mixture of tissues found in the lung, particularly cartilage.

Patients are often symptom-free and a hamartoma is usually discovered on chest X-ray. It is frequently surgically removed as it is difficult to distinguish it from peripheral bronchial carcinoma or tuberculoma.

DISEASES OF THE PLEURA

Pleurisy

Inflammation of the pleura may be *dry* or associated with *effusion*, the former often proceeding to the latter.

Dry Pleurisy

Dry pleurisy may be caused by: tuberculosis which rapidly progresses to pleurisy with effusion; pneumonia or lung abscess; pulmonary infarct; injury to lungs or pleura; rarely in the terminal stages of uraemia. Occasionally primary pleurisy may occur without underlying disease.

CLINICAL FEATURES

The main symptom is a sharp and stabbing pain over the affected area, aggravated by coughing and deep breathing. The respirations may be short and grunting and chest movement limited on the affected side. The diagnosis is confirmed by the presence of a pleural rub. The pain diminishes as an effusion forms.

The chest X-ray may reveal underlying disease, if present, but otherwise shows no specific sign of dry pleurisy.

TREATMENT

Bed rest and treatment of the underlying condition will be required. Analgesics and local heat may be of help in relieving pain, but due regard must be paid to the underlying condition. The patient should be nursed in a position that is most comfortable for his breathing and may choose to lie on the affected side.

179

Pleural Effusion

An accumulation of fluid in the pleural cavity may represent a transudate or an exudate.

TRANSUDATES

These occur when the venous pressure is high or the osmotic pressure of the plasma is reduced. The fluid is usually clear and of low specific gravity and contains less than 2·0 g protein per 100 ml.

Causes of pleural transudates are cardiac failure, the nephrotic syndrome and cirrhosis of the liver.

EXUDATES

These occur in the presence of inflammation or neoplasm. The fluid is of high specific gravity and contains more than 2·0 g protein per 100 ml. Exudates may be clear or cloudy; they will be clear in tuberculous or neoplastic disease but cloudiness may be due to the presence of blood as in neoplasm or pulmonary infarct, or pus cells as in pneumonia or lung abscess.

Causes of pleural exudates are: bacterial pneumonias; pulmonary infarction; secondary pleural malignancy or rarely, a primary tumour such as diffuse malignant mesothelioma; tuberculosis; subphrenic abscess and other complicating inflammatory lesions; collagen disorders; fungal infections. There are also very rare causes such as the postmyocardial syndrome, acute pancreatitis, Meig's syndrome.

TYPICAL SIGNS OF PLEURAL EFFUSION

There is diminished movement on the affected side. If the effusion is large, there may be mediastinal shift to the opposite side. Tactile vocal fremitus is diminished over the fluid. On percussion there is stony dullness over the fluid, the line tending to rise in the axilla with moderate effusions. On auscultation there are absent breath sounds and voice sounds over the fluid. Sometimes bronchial breathing occurs above the upper level of the fluid.

TREATMENT

The pleural reaction which is frequently associated with *bacterial pneumonias* may progress to pleural effusion and should always be suspected if fever persists despite appropriate antibiotics. These effusions should always be aspirated to dryness at once. The fluid is amber or straw-coloured.

Pleural involvement in *pulmonary infarction* is almost invariable and pleural pain is a constant clinical feature. Pleural effusion commonly develops, small to moderate in size. Aspiration is seldom required, but if performed the fluid may be blood-stained but is more commonly clear and straw-coloured.

Primary pleural neoplasm is rare but *secondary pleural malignancy* is common. They have two characteristics, the fluid is often blood-stained and it recurs promptly after aspiration. The patient must be kept comfortable by repeated aspiration; it is sometimes possible to slow down the re-accumulation of fluid by radiotherapy or chemotherapy, but on the whole results are disappointing.

Pleural effusion is commonly associated with primary tuberculosis. The onset is variable, sometimes it is acute with fever, malaise, sweating and severe pleuritic pain as in pleurisy. Other patients may have little pain but complain of vague ill-health and dyspnoea on effort. Treatment will be by means of aspiration and the use of anti-tuberculous drugs. It is important to prevent the development of pleural fibrosis.

Pleural effusion associated with subphrenic abscess should be promptly aspirated and appropriate antibiotic therapy instituted. Surgery may be necessary.

Pleural effusion may occur in association with collagen disorders, fungal infections and other rare disease. Management will consist of treatment of the underlying condition.

PHYSIOTHERAPY

Physiotherapy has no part to play in the treatment of dry pleurisy, transudates or malignant pleural effusion.

Following aspiration of other types of pleural effusion, breathing exercises should be started in order to prevent chest deformity and loss of respiratory function due to thickening of the pleura.

The patient should be given localized expansion exercises to all areas of the affected side; attention should be paid to the apical area even though the effusion is usually in the posterior basal area. Belt exercises are often helpful and the patient should be encouraged to practise several times a day.

If chest movement does not improve, the patient should lie on his unaffected side with two pillows under his thorax in order to open out the ribs on the affected side. He should take up this position for half an hour at a time at least four times a day and should be encouraged to practise intermittent expansion exercises whilst in this position.

Treatment should be continued until chest expansion is equal and the X-ray has improved.

EMPYEMA

This is a localized collection of pus in the pleural cavity. It is most commonly a complication of lobar pneumonia but it may also be associated with bronchiectasis or due to spread of infection from a lung abscess, subphrenic abscess, mediastinal sepsis, a chest wound or a complication of thoracic surgery. It may also result from a tuberculous infection of the pleural cavity.

CLINICAL FEATURES

Empyema most commonly occurs one to two weeks after the start of a pneumococcal pneumonia. Instead of the normal process of recovery, the patient remains ill, the temperature begins to rise again and is of a remittent character accompanied by drenching sweats; there is general malaise and anorexia.

Examination of the chest reveals signs of fluid, *i.e.* dullness to percussion and absent or diminished breath sounds over the area; in children there may be bronchial breathing over the area which may lead to the erroneous diagnosis of unresolved pneumonia.

Postero-anterior and lateral X-rays will reveal the locality of the fluid and diagnosis will be confirmed by aspiration. In the early stages of empyema the fluid is thin and serous but in the later stages it becomes thick and purulent. The aspirated fluid should be cultured for organisms. Fluid may become loculated and difficult to aspirate.

PROGNOSIS

With correct treatment, the prognosis for empyema is good.

TREATMENT

The aims of treatment are control of infection, removal of pus and obliteration of the empyema space.

In the early stages of empyema, the infected pleural effusion must be aspirated daily and an appropriate antibiotic should be injected into the pleural cavity. An antibiotic should also be given orally or parenterally. These measures will usually result in a cure. In the case of tuberculous empyema, antituberculous drugs will be given.

If this treatment is not effective, the aspirated fluid will become thick and purulent and a chronic empyema will develop. In this case, surgical intervention will be necessary by means of a decortication or drainage by rib resection (see page 210).

Physiotherapy will be on the same lines as for pleural effusion, although chest deformity is more likely to occur and recovery will be slower.

Pre- and post-operative treatment may be required (see page 181).

HAEMOTHORAX

Haemothorax usually follows trauma to the chest wall, but it may also be associated with pneumothorax, when it is known as haemo-pneumothorax. Occasionally an aneurysm may rupture into the pleural cavity and cause a haemothorax.

Blood in the pleural cavity clots rapidly and fibrin will be deposited on the pleural surfaces. Pleural reaction will occur with further out-pouring of fluid. If blood is left in the pleural cavity, pleural fibrosis occurs which will result in serious interference with lung function.

CLINICAL FEATURES

If pleural bleeding is excessive, the patient will be shocked and collapsed, with rapid pulse and respiration. There may not be external evidence of trauma but there will be signs of fluid in the chest. Diagnosis will be confirmed by aspiration of blood from the pleural cavity. It is important to distinguish between the presence of haemorrhage and blood-stained pleural effusion.

TREATMENT

General treatment for internal haemorrhage should be given. The effusion should be aspirated daily in order to keep the pleural space as dry as possible. Antibiotics should be given at this stage as there is danger of secondary infection.

Surgical intervention may be necessary in cases of severe bleeding or damage to the chest wall, or if the blood cannot be evacuated by aspiration.

Physiotherapy will be as for pleural effusion once the haemorrhage has been controlled.

SPONTANEOUS PNEUMOTHORAX

A collection of air in the pleural cavity as a result of a pathological process is known as a spontaneous pneumothorax.

Spontaneous pneumothorax most commonly occurs in young males and is caused by the rupture of a bleb under the visceral pleura. It is thought these blebs are caused by a congenital defect in the alveolar wall.

It may also complicate lung disease such as asthma, emphysema, pulmonary tuberculosis, congenital cysts, cystic fibrosis, lung abscess and pneumoconiosis. Air in the pleural cavity may also be caused by wounds, perforation of the oesophagus or trachea, or following thoracic surgery.

When a spontaneous pneumothorax occurs as the result of a ruptured bleb, the leak usually seals off rapidly and air in the pleural cavity absorbs in a week or so. Occasionally a valve-like leak occurs and air will enter the pleural cavity on inspiration but is unable to escape on expiration; this leads to an accumulation of air and is known as a *tension pneumothorax*.

CLINICAL FEATURES

Onset is usually sudden and is associated with pain on the affected side of the chest and dyspnoea. It is occasionally precipitated by a sudden movement. The degree of distress suffered varies according to the size of the pneumothorax and the condition of the lungs.

On examination, the chest movement will be diminished on the affected side. There will be mediastinal displacement away from the affected side, the degree varying according to the size of the pneumothorax. The percussion note is either normal or hyper-resonant. There will be diminished breath sounds over the site of the pneumothorax.

The development of a *tension pneumothorax* will be indicated by increasing dyspnoea, cyanosis and distress. There will be signs of a pneumothorax with considerable mediastinal displacement. Measures to relieve the tension must be taken immediately, otherwise death may occur.

The chest X-ray will show air in the pleural cavity with a varying amount of lung collapse.

TREATMENT

When a spontaneous pneumothorax has been diagnosed shortly after onset, it is wiser to admit the patient to hospital as there is always a risk of tension pneumothorax or haemopneumothorax developing.

If there is a large pneumothorax or if the patient is in great distress, a needle should be inserted into the pleural space and the pressure recorded; if a tension pneumothorax has occurred the pressure will become positive instead of negative. It is often necessary to insert a pleural drain connected to an under-water seal, then expansion of the lung will usually take place within a day or so. If expansion fails to take place, or if the pneumothorax recurs, it may be necessary to consider pleurodesis (the induction of chemical pleurisy) or pleurectomy (see page 209).

If the pneumothorax is very small, the patient should rest in bed for a few days and re-expansion will probably occur without further measures being taken.

Physiotherapy is contra-indicated in the early treatment of spontaneous pneumothorax. Once a drainage tube has been inserted, breathing exercises may be ordered to obtain full re-expansion of the lung and expansion exercises should be given to all areas of the affected side. Full range arm movements should also be given.

If pleurodesis is carried out the patient will have a severe pleural reaction and breathing exercises should be started the day after introduction of the irritant substance into the pleural cavity. Treatment will be on the same lines as for pleural effusion but the patient is often in a great deal of pain and it is helpful to administer an analgesic before treatment is attempted. A drainage tube is often inserted and arm exercises should also be given.

If pleurectomy is to be carried out, pre- and post-operative physiotherapy will be necessary (see page 210).

REFERENCES

Miller, G. A. H. & Sutton, G. C. (1970). 'Massive Pulmonary Embolism.' *British Journal of Hospital Medicine*, June 1970 issue.

Oswald, N. C., Hinson, K. F. W., Canti, G. & Miller, A. A. (1971).'The Diagnosis of Primary Lung Cancer with Special Reference to Sputum Cytology.' *Thorax*, No. 26, 623.

BIBLIOGRAPHY
(Chapters 5–8)

Basmajian, J. M. (1971). *Grant's Method of Anatomy*. The Williams and Wilkins Co., Baltimore. 8th ed.

Bates, D. V., Macklem, P. T. & Christie, R. V. (1971). *Respiratory Function in Disease*. W. B. Saunders Co., Philadelphia, London, Toronto.

Brompton Hospital (1967). *Physiotherapy for Medical and Surgical Thoracic Conditions*. London.

Campbell, E. J. M., Agostoni, E. & Newsom Davis, J. (1970). *The Respiratory Muscles—Mechanics and Neural Control*. Lloyd-Luke (Medical Books) Ltd., London.

Chest and Heart Association (1964). *Cystic Fibrosis*. London.

Comroe, J. H., Forster, R. E., Dubois, A. B., Briscoe, W. A. & Carlson, E. (1970). *The Lung*. Year Book Medical Publishers Inc., Chicago.

Crofton, J. & Douglas, A. (1969). *Respiratory Diseases*. Blackwell, Oxford and Edinburgh.

Gaskell, D. V. & Webber, B. A. (1973). *The Brompton Hospital Guide to Chest Physiotherapy*. Blackwell, Oxford.

Houston, J. C., Joiner, C. L. & Trounce, J. R. (1970). *A Short Textbook of Medicine*. English Universities Press, London.

Last, R. J. (1972). *Anatomy—Regional and Applied*. Churchill-Livingstone, Edinburgh. 5th ed.

Reid, Lynne (1967). *The Pathology of Emphysema*. Lloyd-Luke (Medical Books) Ltd., London.

Sykes, M. K., McNicol, M. W. & Campbell, E. J. M. (1970). *Respiratory Failure*. Blackwell, Oxford and Edinburgh.

Thacker, E. W. (1971). *Postural Drainage and Respiratory Control*. Lloyd-Luke (Medical Books) Ltd., London.

CHAPTER 9

Thoracic Surgery—I

by D. M. INNOCENTI, M.C.S.P.

INTRODUCTION

The importance of physiotherapy in the surgical treatment of chest conditions has been gradually accepted and is now firmly established. In the early years, radical surgical treatment for tuberculosis often resulted in severe deformity. More recently much surgical progress has been made, including perfection of lung resections and open heart surgery. Concurrently, physiotherapeutic techniques have advanced and expanded, helping to make it possible for patients to return to fully active lives.

INCISIONS USED IN THORACIC SURGERY

The direction of the thoracic incision may be:
1. Oblique   —lateral
2. Transverse }
3. Vertical   } —anterior

Lateral Incisions

Thoracotomy. The standard unilateral method of entry into the thorax is through an intercostal space. The level of entry depends entirely on the area on which the operation is to be performed. The incision runs antero-laterally or postero-laterally (see Fig. 9/1). The former divides the lower fibres of pectoralis major, serratus anterior, and the external and internal intercostals, terminating at the anterior border of the latissimus dorsi. The latter divides the lower fibres of trapezius, latissimus dorsi, serratus anterior and the external and

187

internal intercostals. A high posterior continuation of the incision also divides the rhomboid major and the erector spinae.

Anterior Incisions

For operations on the heart or mediastinum the approach is usually from the front.

a) The transverse approach is submammary and bilateral (see Fig. 9/1), through the fourth intercostal spaces and a transversely divided

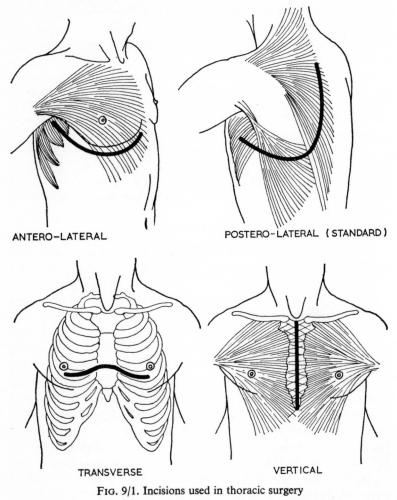

ANTERO–LATERAL   POSTERO–LATERAL (STANDARD)

TRANSVERSE   VERTICAL

FIG. 9/1. Incisions used in thoracic surgery

sternum. The pectoralis major is divided together with the external and internal intercostals.

ᶦb) The vertical approach. Median sternotomy is probably the most commonly used anterior incision (see Fig. 9/1). The sternum is divided longitudinally and retracted. No muscles are divided but the action of the pectoralis major is affected because the pre-sternal aponeurosis is cut. A cosmetic incision is sometimes preferred for children or women. It is Y-shaped with the limbs of the Y at the third intercostal space.

The level of the incision and the muscles divided will determine the post-operative postural programme. Pain and abnormal muscle pull will create post-operative faults with possible deformity and limitation of movement.

The thoracotomy incision sometimes creates a scoliosis towards the operation side, *i.e.* a low shoulder and a high hip. The thoracoplasty operation (see page 211) produces the opposite deformity. Due to loss of structural support the patient leans away from the affected side and compensates with a cervical shift towards the incision. Latissimus dorsi, the rhomboids, serratus anterior, trapezius and pectoralis major all exert forces on the scapula and the humerus, thus compromising shoulder movements.

DRAINAGE

Drainage of unwanted fluid and air from the thorax is necessary following both surgery and/or other trauma. Drainage may be a) closed or b) open.

a) Closed drainage. To allow drainage from the thorax but simultaneously prevent air entry, a simple air-tight system is used. A rubber or plastic tube with end and side holes is introduced into the thorax through an intercostal space and fixed with a purse-string suture. It is connected to a closed calibrated drainage bottle via a glass tube which terminates under water (see Fig. 9/2). Another short glass tube passes through the rubber bung of the bottle to allow free drainage, or to allow connection to a suction pump which aids drainage. Air and fluid will pass down the tube. The patency of the tube must be maintained by frequent attention and 'milking' to prevent or remove clots.

b) Open drainage is occasionally used to drain thickened and infected matter from an empyema cavity. An area of infection, which

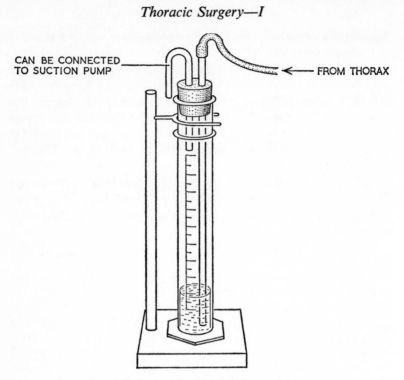

CAN BE CONNECTED
TO SUCTION PUMP

FROM THORAX

Fig. 9/2. System for closed drainage of thorax

is localized by fibrosis from the remaining pleura, renders it impossible to create a pneumothorax. Pus and debris track down the tube or corrugated drain into a dressing.

On free drainage the level of the fluid in the glass tube will be seen to rise on inspiration and fall on expiration, due to the alteration in intrathoracic pressure. Bubbles denote escape of air and these increase on coughing. If the fluid level ceases to swing it means either that the tubing is blocked or that the lung is fully expanded. The fluid level should *not* swing when on suction because the air pressure in the bottle is lower than the intrathoracic pressure.

The drainage bottle must at all times remain at a lower level than the patient to prevent siphoning of fluid back into the chest. Clamping of the tubes may be necessary during difficult changes of position, but it is not necessary for the patient to remain in bed during the drainage period.

Intercostal or subcostal drainage tubes are used to drain:

190

1. Pleural cavity.
   a) apical—mainly air
   b) basal —mainly fluid.
2. Mediastinum.
3. Pericardial space.

PRE-OPERATIVE PERIOD
Investigations

Before surgery patients will undergo extensive investigations. All patients have chest X-rays, respiratory function tests (see page 40), dental examinations, sputum culture, haematological investigations and electrocardiographic studies.

Patients with respiratory disease will possibly also undergo further tests as follows:

BRONCHOSCOPY

This procedure entails introducing a bronchoscope via the mouth to allow direct examination of the larynx, trachea, carina and the main bronchi and bronchial orifices. Suction and biopsy may be carried out during the examination.

BRONCHOGRAPHY

This is a radiographic examination in which a radio-opaque substance is introduced into the bronchial tree by means of a naso-tracheal catheter or by direct injection into the trachea. The airways are outlined and any distortion, obstruction, stricture or dilation demonstrated. The resulting radiograph is of particular interest to the physiotherapist in cases of bronchiectasis, as the affected areas are minutely delineated. Physiotherapy and postural drainage is essential prior to the investigation to clear excess secretions from the bronchial tree.

The patient should not eat or drink for approximately two hours after the examination, since the larynx has been anaesthetized and fluid may enter the lungs.

Patients with cardiac lesions may undergo the following investigations:

CARDIAC CATHETERIZATION

This examination is performed under local anaesthesia. A catheter is introduced into the right side of the heart through the venous system commencing at the median cubital vein. The tricuspid and pulmonary valves are traversed and the catheter finally lodged into the pulmonary arteries. The left side of the heart and the aortic and mitral valves are examined. The catheter is introduced into the femoral artery and passed retrogradely in the aorta.

Pressures within the chambers and vessels, and pressure gradients across the valves, are measured and oxygen saturation studies are made. The cardiac output may be calculated from oxygen saturation measurements. The diagnosis of congenital abnormalities is also confirmed by catheterization.

ANGIOCARDIOGRAPHY AND ANGIOGRAPHY

These are radiographic studies following the injection of contrast media into the heart and/or vessels to demonstrate irregularities, blockages, constrictions and aneurysms.

Patient Assessment

The physiotherapist must become conversant with the patient's history, and examination should take account of the following:

1. Shape of chest. Deformities may be a) congenital or b) acquired.

a) Some congenital deformities affecting the thorax are: scoliosis; kyphosis; pectus carinatum (pigeon chest)—the middle portion of the sternum and the adjoining ribs protrude; pectus excavatum (funnel chest)—the lower one-third of the sternum is depressed and the ribs cave inwards to form a hollow.

b) Some acquired deformities are: barrel chest—chest held high in inspiratory position with an increased anteroposterior diameter; scoliosis or kyphosis—may be idiopathic or be secondary to disease, trauma or operation; asymmetry—due to rib flattening and impaired movement.

2. Movements of respiration.

a) Thoracic upper costal } unilateral or
„ lower costal } bilateral

b) Diaphragmatic.

3. Signs of cardiopulmonary insufficiency. a) cyanosis; b) clubbing of fingers and toes; c) oedema of the ankles; d) raised jugular venous pressure (if present note whether it is sustained or whether it falls on inspiration); e) dyspnoea; f) orthopnoea.

4. Sputum. Note a) the type—mucoid; mucopurulent; bloody; b) the quantity; c) the viscosity.

5. Joint movements. Range of movement of thoracic spine, neck, shoulder girdle and shoulders must be ascertained.

6. Exercise tolerance. The distance and speed at which the patient is able to walk must be established: a) on the level; b) on slopes and c) on stairs.

7. Special investigations. All relevant data must be examined. The X-ray should be studied in order to compare it with the post-operative condition. Respiratory function results must be considered. The vital capacity and forced expiratory volume in one second is of special importance when lung resection is contemplated. Broncho-scopy, bronchogram, cardiac catheterization and angiographic results should be examined.

8. Cerebral function. It must be appreciated that there are some definite relationships between cardiac disease and cerebrovascular accidents.

a) Atherosclerosis is a generalized disease and is the underlying cause of angina pectoris, cerebrovascular disease and intermittent claudication.

b) Emboli are frequently thrown off diseased heart valves, resulting in cerebrovascular accidents.

c) There is a definite incidence of intracranial berry aneurysm formation occurring when there is coarctation of the aorta.

Principles of Physiotherapy

1. To explain and teach post-operative procedures: a) breathing exercises; b) arm, leg and general exercises; and c) postural awareness.

2. To teach awareness of breathing and relationships of thoracic, diaphragmatic and air movements.

3. To mobilize thoracic cage by: a) general rib movements; b) bilateral and unilateral localized rib movements; c) trunk and shoulder girdle exercises.

4. To increase diaphragm excursion and control by localized diaphragmatic breathing exercises.

G   193

5. To clear secretions by: a) cough; b) postural drainage, per-cussion and shakings; c) inhalation therapy; d) intermittent positive pressure breathing.

Techniques of Physiotherapy

POSITIONS OF THE PATIENT AND THE PHYSIOTHERAPIST FOR BREATHING INSTRUCTION
The patient's position is important in order to achieve relaxation, concentration and freedom of thoracic and abdominal movement.

The positions for the initial instructions are: a) half-lying; b) side-lying with upper arm (and possibly upper leg) supported on a pillow; c) high side-lying with the arm supported on a pillow; d) sitting in a comfortable upright chair.

Although unorthodox, it is more efficient for the physiotherapist to sit on the side of the bed when the patient is in the half-lying position. This facilitates communication with the patient and obser-vation and control of the thorax and abdomen.

When the patient is sitting in a chair the physiotherapist should sit facing and to the side of him. With the patient in either of the side-lying positions the physiotherapist should stand *behind* him. This affords an unobstructed view of the patient's face and lessens the risk of cross-infection from sputum. The therapist is unencum-bered by the patient's arms when controlling the thorax and abdomen and in helping him to alter position.

BREATHING EXERCISES
Very often patients are quite unaware of the relationships between thoracic and abdominal movements and air flow. A short explanation of these mechanics should be given and these factors kept in mind by the patient and the physiotherapist, as increased movement does *not* always mean increased function.

When the patient is aware of these respiratory and air movements during quiet breathing, and relaxed (it may be necessary to use the contrast method of relaxation), attention is directed towards the specific exercises. Although costal and diaphragmatic movements occur simultaneously they must be considered separately for treat-ment purposes.

Thoracic cage movements. Costal movements can be localized to the following areas and can be practised bilaterally and unilaterally, where necessary: i) apices; ii) lower lateral costal; iii) posterior basal (see Fig. 9/3).

In the past much emphasis has been placed on localized movements, but practice is now moving towards a more general pattern of movement. There is very little information on whether or not localized rib movement produces an underlying localized lung expansion. However, these exercises do have value where there is localized diminution of movement due to underlying disease or to pain.

COSTAL EXERCISES

The exercises are best taught by instruction in one phase at a time, progressing to the full cycle. Air flow and movement must both be referred to, and manual resistance given on inspiration. In some cases assistance may be given at the end of expiration.

Inspiratory and expansion exercises are practised by concentrating on a gentle but full inspiration and expansion of the ribs against the physiotherapist's hands, which are placed firmly on the chest wall to guide and facilitate movement. An initial intercostal stretch may be given, followed by moderate pressure as the patient tries to expand the desired area and hold the breath for a few seconds on full inspiration. Encouragement is given verbally and manually. Resistance is gradually released during expiration, which ceases at the resting point of the thorax and abdomen. The expiratory phase is not emphasized at this stage. The exercise is continued until good, easy movement and air flow are achieved.

Expiratory costal exercises. The object is maximum costal movement and expiration, to stimulate and encourage coughing. The patient tries to breathe out fully but gently, using active contraction of expiratory muscles. The physiotherapist may assist by increasing the manual pressure at the point of maximum expiration before minimally resisting the ensuing inspiration. Full expiratory exercises are a useful precursor to coughing. Full range costal breathing exercises may soon tire the patient and produce an unpleasant giddiness if protracted.

DIAPHRAGMATIC BREATHING

There is some diversity of opinion on the teaching of diaphragmatic breathing. Basically there are two schools of thought. One concen-

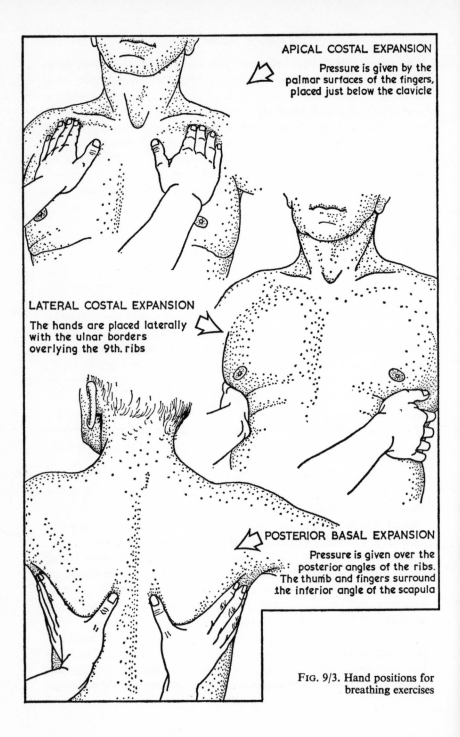

APICAL COSTAL EXPANSION
Pressure is given by the palmar surfaces of the fingers, placed just below the clavicle

LATERAL COSTAL EXPANSION
The hands are placed laterally with the ulnar borders overlying the 9th. ribs

POSTERIOR BASAL EXPANSION
Pressure is given over the posterior angles of the ribs. The thumb and fingers surround the inferior angle of the scapula

FIG. 9/3. Hand positions for breathing exercises

trates on epigastric and lower rib movement (swelling of the epigastrium and widening the costal angle). The other concentrates on
allowing the whole abdomen to swell as the diaphragm descends (see
Fig. 9/4). The writer advocates the latter technique, since it is much
easier for the patient to learn and is at least as effective.

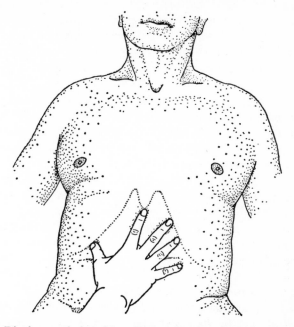

Fig. 9/4. Diaphragmatic breathing. Slight resistance to diaphragmatic descent
during inspiration is given with the hand over the abdomen, the fingers extending
into the sub-costal angle

Diaphragmatic breathing is now widely taught by placing the
whole hand on the abdomen (if the patient is very large both hands
may be necessary). Gentle resistance is given to the abdominal wall
during inspiration and the patient is instructed to allow his abdomen
to swell, gently not forcibly, as he breathes in. During expiration
resistance should not be reduced suddenly, rather the weight of the
hand should follow the abdomen back to the resting position.

When costal and diaphragmatic breathing exercises are mastered
they should be practised in the side-lying or high side-lying position.
The unilateral thoracic movement (the upper hemithorax) will be
controlled by the physiotherapist's hands on the anterior and posterior

aspects of the thorax. The diaphragmatic movement will be controlled and resisted by placing a hand, or hands, on the abdomen. The breathing exercises must be practised to gain control and confidence. If there is sufficient time pre-operatively, the instruction of alteration in depth and pace of breathing, and synchronization of walking and breathing, will help very distressed patients. The synchronization of walking and breathing can be practised in two ways, by (i) the counting method, for instance taking two steps during inspiration and three steps for expiration, (ii) consciously maintaining a regular breathing rhythm.

'*Huffing*' is a breathing exercise designed as a precursor to coughing. There are two methods:

a) A deep inspiration is taken and the expiratory phase is broken into a series of short sharp 'pants', the procedure being controlled mainly by the abdominal muscles.

b) Shallow breaths, in and out, through the mouth, gradually gaining depth and strength, are controlled by general costal movements.

The irregular air flow, resulting from either method, loosens sputum and eases it towards the larger bronchi, whence it can be cleared by a cough.

REMOVAL OF BRONCHIAL SECRETIONS

Coughing is essential to maintain patency of the airways and their dependent alveoli. In the healthy lung, secretions are continuously moved upwards by the action of the ciliated epithelium lining the main airways. In damaged lung this action is diminished or absent. Conscious coughing must therefore be taught and practised.

A considerable amount of air must be inspired quickly, and the glottis and vocal cords closed. (Patients suffering from recurrent laryngeal nerve palsy have great difficulty in coughing.) Simultaneous contractions of all the expiratory muscles of the abdomen and the thorax generate a high intrapulmonary pressure. On opening the glottis an explosive jet of air issues from the trachea, carrying with it any foreign matter. Since a high intrathoracic pressure obstructs the flow of blood to the heart, a prolonged bout of coughing may cause the cardiac output to fall and the patient may faint (cough syncope). Patients must be taught to avoid this by controlling their cough and doing no more than three to five coughs on one breath.

198

Cough holds. The patient must understand the importance of coughing and be assured that it will do no damage post-operatively. To ease the obviously painful manoeuvre he should be taught how to stabilize his chest when coughing alone.

The thoracotomy incision is best supported by placing the hand of the unaffected side as far round the affected ribs as possible and applying firm pressure with the hand and forearm. The other hand reinforces the hugging hold by clasping the opposite elbow and pulling it against the chest wall during the cough. The anterior thoracic incisions will best be supported by holding both hands across the sternum.

Vibrations. Should it not be possible to clear the lungs adequately by breathing exercises and coughing, percussion, vibrations and shakings may be necessary. Percussion must be avoided in the following instances: a) acute pneumonia; b) acute lung abscess; c) neoplasms; d) haemoptysis.

Attention should be directed to one hemithorax at a time. Vibrations and shaking are most effective if they are administered with the hands on the posterior and anterior aspects of the hemithorax and the shakings directed towards an internal focal point.

Postural drainage. The positions are shown on page 115 *et seq.*

Inhalation therapy. This may be used in conjunction with physiotherapy in the following situations:

1. For sputum liquefaction. Substances available are: a) Alevaire (a detergent); b) Airbron (acetylcysteine, which breaks the disulphide bonds in mucus); c) Ascoxal (a mixture which depolymerizes the polysaccharide molecule in mucus).

2. For the relief of bronchospasm: a) Isoprenaline sulphate (which is also a cardiac stimulant); b) Alupent (which is also a cardiac stimulant); c) Ventolin (salbutamol) is now widely used as it has minimal cardiovascular effects.

3. For topical treatment: a) antibiotics; b) fungicides.

The finest particles of moisture for inhalation are produced by nebulizers and sometimes inhalation is assisted by intermittent positive pressure breathing (I.P.P.B.) (see page 128 *et seq.*).

Drug therapy. Systemic therapy may be instituted to lessen the viscosity of mucoid sputum. *Bisolvon* is such a mucolytic agent and may be administered orally in tablet or elixir form.

GENERAL EXERCISES

Individual instruction in leg exercises should be given pre-operatively, in the lying and half-lying positions. The head and neck, shoulder girdle, arm and trunk exercises will best be taught in a class, along with postural awareness and correction. A close watch must be kept to avoid undue fatigue, especially of the cardiac patients who are fit enough to take part. Many cardiac patients should not join these exercise sessions.

Guide to a typical ward class for pre-operative and post-operative respiratory and cardiac patients.

On the first post-operative day patients in bed will attempt the neck and shoulder girdle movements, breathing and foot exercises. Trunk exercises are added about the third post-operative day. Preoperative and fourth day post-operative patients should attempt all the exercises.

The scheme of exercises will include:

Deep bilateral costal breathing in time with instructor.
Head and neck rotation, flexion and extension.
Shoulder shrugging and bracing.
Arms bend and stretch forwards, sideways and upwards.
Diaphragmatic breathing in own time.
Foot and ankle exercises.
Alternate hip and knee flexion and extension.
Arms stretch sideways and place alternately behind neck and waist.
Trunk flexion to alternate sides.
Trunk forward flexion and extension.
Arms bend and circle elbows.
Lateral costal breathing in own time.
Trunk rotation to alternate sides with arms swinging.
Arms stretch out to sides and flex and rotate trunk to touch alternate
    hand to opposite foot.
Postural correction.
Diaphragmatic breathing in time with instructor.

POST-OPERATIVE PERIOD

Principles of Physiotherapy

1. To expand lung tissue by maximum inspiratory efforts with ribs and diaphragm.

2. To prevent lung collapse and/or consolidation by: a) general

and localized costal and diaphragmatic breathing exercises; b) vibrations, shakings and postural drainage; c) coughing.

3. To remove excess secretions by: a) increasing rib and diaphragmatic movement; b) altering volume and speed of air flow; c) shaking, vibrations, percussion and postural drainage; d) coughing; e) suction.

4. To prevent circulatory complications by: a) foot and leg movements; b) general movements; c) deep breathing.

5. To maintain or increase mobility of thorax, head, neck, shoulder girdle and arms by: a) passive movements (for unconscious patients); b) active assisted movements; c) active movements; d) posture correction.

6. To return the patient to as full and as independent a life as possible.

A rope tied to the foot of the bed and extending to the fold of the bed-clothes aids independent movements. Most thoracic units encourage patients to dress fully as soon as all intercostal tubes are removed and to walk freely around the ward and grounds.

Patient Assessment

The physiotherapist must note:
- a) The operation performed.
- b) The incision.
- c) Drainage tubes:
  - i) number and position
  - ii) amount and type of drainage.
- d) Other tubes *in situ*:
  - i) Ryle's tube
  - ii) urethral catheter
  - iii) intravenous lines
  - iv) arterial lines
  - v) endotracheal tube
  - vi) tracheostomy tube.
- e) Temperature.
- f) Pulse.
- g) Respiration:
  - i) spontaneous—rate and depth
  - ii) artificial—rate, pressure and volume.
- h) Blood pressure.

i) Drugs prescribed, especially the type and time of administration of analgesics. Treatment ideally is timed to coincide with analgesic times as pain inhibits breathing and coughing.
j) E.C.G. pattern.
k) X-ray.
l) Blood gases.

Post-operative Cough Holds

The physiotherapist can assist the coughing manoeuvre greatly by her encouragement and manual support.

The thoracotomy incision can best be supported in the lying, half-lying, or side-lying positions by firm pressure of the physiotherapist's hands on the anterior and posterior aspects of the affected side of the thorax. Probably the forward-sitting position is the most effective for coughing, and the physiotherapist should stand on the unaffected side of the patient. The anterior and posterior aspects of the affected side of the thorax can be supported with the hands, whilst at the same time the forearms will stabilize the whole chest and create a 'bear hug' hold.

The median sternotomy should be stabilized by placing both hands on the anterior aspect of the chest, one on each side, and the fingers parallel to the sternum. Equal pressures must be exerted to minimize sternal movement.

Post-operative Complications

Post-operative shock, or excessively low blood pressure, is uncommon nowadays, due to adequate fluid transfusion and administration of vasopressor agents. It might occur, should there be a secondary haemorrhage.

Collapse and/or consolidation of segments or lobes of the lung are due to: a) excessive production of secretions; b) function of cilia being compromised by anaesthesia and surgical intervention; c) excessive fluid or air in the pleural cavity; d) inhibition of cough due to pain and fear; e) diminished respiratory movements; f) infection.

Cardiac arrythmia is due to surgical interference, diminished blood supply, electrolytic imbalance or anoxia.

Carbon dioxide retention is due to inadequate ventilation.

Hypoxia may be due to ventilation/perfusion imbalance, inade quate ventilation, or both.

Deep vein thrombosis. Factors leading to deep vein thrombosis include venous stagnation, rise in platelets secondary to operation, trauma and dehydration. Movement would seem to prevent their formation. However, patients who are ambulant from the first post-operative day are still at risk. Recent work shows that prevention is only possible if blood flow is aided locally whilst the patient is on the operating table. Daily examination of the calf is necessary for early diagnosis.

Pulmonary emboli may be thrown off from a deep vein thrombosis.

Cerebrovascular accident. Emboli may be thrown off from calcified or fungoid heart valves. After cardiopulmonary by-pass the incidence of recurring cerebrovascular insufficiency in patients with previous cerebral damage is high.

Surgical emphysema is the collection of air in the interstitial spaces of subcutaneous tissues. On examination the chest, and possibly also the neck and face, appear swollen. On palpation the tissues crackle and the air can be moved under the fingers. On X-ray the tissues have a mottled appearance due to the air bubbles.

Infections may occur at any of the following sites: i) superficial incision; ii) sternum (post-sternotomy); iii) pleura; iv) mediastinum; v) pericardium.

Pleural effusions are due to secondary haemorrhage, infection or exudation (see page 180). If excessive, aspiration or drainage with an intercostal tube will be necessary.

Pericardial effusions after surgery are usually due to haemorrhage. If the pericardium is left open the fluid will not restrict the heart's action. *Cardiac tamponade:* should the pericardium be intact the collection of fluid within the non-elastic sac could be fatal. Fluid collecting in the pericardial cavity prevents the heart from filling during diastole. Hence cardiac output and blood pressure fall. Cardiac arrest will supervene unless emergency measures are taken and the thorax entered to incise the pericardium.

Ventilatory arrest is usually the result of total occlusion of the airway by mucus, or a foreign body.

Cardiac arrest may be total asystole or due to ventricular fibrillation (see page 255).

Restricted arm and trunk movements may lead to an acquired-deformity.

Renal complications occasionally precede acute failure and may necessitate peritoneal or haemodialysis.

Post bypass syndrome may complicate the recovery period. The patient feels unwell, lethargic and has a swinging pyrexia. It may be due to a pericardial and pleural reaction and is usually successfully treated with a three-day course of aspirin or steroid therapy.

Bronchopleural fistula may occur by breakdown of the bronchial stump or lung tissue. Air will pass directly from the bronchus into the pleural cavity and create or increase a pneumothorax. Bronchopleural fistula in pneumonectomy—see page 207.

For references and bibliography, see end of Chapter 11.

CHAPTER 10

Thoracic Surgery—II

by D. M. INNOCENTI, M.C.S.P.

OPERATIONS ON LUNG TISSUE

Local Resections

Local lesions of bronchiectasis, tuberculosis, neoplasms, benign tumours, fungus infections, hydatid, congenital or emphysematous cysts may be resected from the lung tissue. The standard thoracotomy incision is used for: a) *wedge resection*—a local resection; b) *segmental resection*—removal of a bronchopulmonary segment; c) *lobectomy*—removal of an entire lobe; d) *sleeve resection*—removal of upper lobe and section of the main bronchus.

It must be established that the patient has sufficient ventilatory reserve to undergo radical excision and survive the first few difficult days. Chronic lung disease may contra-indicate or defer surgery.

The unresected lung tissue expands into the vacant space, thus repositioning the airways. Should postural drainage be necessary the authentic positions may no longer suffice, and individual variants must be found.

PRE-OPERATIVE PHYSIOTHERAPY
This will follow the usual regime. Postural drainage is an important factor when much sputum is present. All patients should join the ward class. Auto-assisted shoulder elevation and the cough hold must be taught.

POST-OPERATIVE PHYSIOTHERAPY
Lateral costal and diaphragmatic breathing exercises and coughing

are commenced on the day of the operation. Full active assisted shoulder elevation and abduction must be gained. Oxygen therapy is administered for the first few hours.

First post-operative day. Foot, leg, arm and shoulder girdle movements should be practised regularly through the day. The patient should be encouraged to expand the remaining lung tissue, by taking deep inspirations and holding each breath for a few seconds at full inspiration.

Resisted inspiratory costal and diaphragmatic breathing exercises, shakings (if necessary) and coughing should begin with the patient in side lying, possibly with the bed tipped. Similar exercises and bilateral costal exercises should next be practised with the patient lying back onto a pillow (quarter turn up from supine). The pillow should be placed along the patient's back and the intercostal tubes arranged to rest over it. This position 'opens up' the anterior chest wall and facilitates bilateral costal movement whilst still draining the affected lung. The breathing exercises should next be repeated in the lying position. The foot of the bed is lowered and all exercises and coughing repeated in half lying.

Second post-operative day. All exercises are increased and trunk movements added to the scheme in the sitting position. The patient may sit out of bed for as long as he wishes. Drainage tubes will probably be removed.

Third post-operative day. The full ward class regime should be attempted.

All exercises and postural drainage must be continued until the lungs are clear and fully expanded. Postural exercises and general activities should be progressed until discharge about the eleventh day. Young people recovering from resections for bronchiectasis need encouragement to play games in the gymnasium or grounds.

Pneumonectomy

The removal of a whole lung is commonly undertaken for excision of a carcinoma and rarely for benign disease. The other lung must be healthy and capable of supporting life. It may be impossible to maintain adequate respiration with one lung if the vital capacity is very low.

The operation may be localized or radical. Radical pneumonectomy includes excision of mediastinal glands and dissection from the chest wall or pericardium. The phrenic and recurrent laryngeal nerves may be involved, resulting in a paralysis of a hemi-diaphragm and inability to approximate the vocal cords. The latter seriously impairs the ability to cough.

Intercostal drainage is rarely used. The hemithorax is filled with fluid and air. The fluid level may need to be controlled by aspirations to prevent submersion of the bronchial stump, or a mediastinal shift. The fluid will finally organize and the hemi-diaphragm rise.

PRE-OPERATIVE PHYSIOTHERAPY

This will follow the usual routine, particular attention being paid to expansion of the base of the remaining lung and to diaphragmatic control.

POST-OPERATIVE PHYSIOTHERAPY

Oxygen therapy is administered for the first few hours. Most surgeons prefer their patients not to turn onto the unaffected side, as the fluid will submerge the bronchial stump. If the bronchial stump breaks down, thus creating a bronchopleural fistula, the fluid would drain across into the remaining lung.

Costal and diaphragmatic exercises for the remaining lung are necessary from the day of operation. *Straining* to cough should be avoided for twenty-four hours. Postural drainage will be included if there is sputum retention. As drainage necessitates lying on the incision the positioning must be carefully executed. The patient should sit forward and then turn into side sitting towards the affected side. The physiotherapist will stand behind the patient and rearrange the pillows, leaving only one on the bed. The patient's body-weight must be supported at the shoulder as he lowers himself on to his elbow and then into side lying.

Although there is only one lung, bilateral costal exercises are important to retain symmetry. Breathing control and exercise tolerance can be improved by the encouragement of diaphragmatic breathing. General exercises are progressed as for a lobectomy. Recovery is often slow, due to age and the gravity of the disease.

Should a bronchopleural fistula occur from breakdown of the bronchial stump, it will be recognized by dyspnoea, irritating cough and possible expectoration of a dark fluid. The patient must sit up or be turned on to the operation side to prevent any spill-over of pleural fluid to the remaining lung.

Infants

Lung resections are rarely undertaken in infants and young children. The most common causes for surgery are as follows:

Congenital intrathoracic cysts may cause acute respiratory distress and will necessitate thoracotomy and excision of the cyst.

Congenital obstructive lobar emphysema occurs occasionally between the ages of one week and two years. The over-inflated lobe compresses the adjacent lung tissue and may also cause a mediastinal shift with subsequent compression of the other lung. The child will become wheezy, dyspnoeic and cyanotic. Thoracotomy will be necessary to perform a lobectomy.

Bronchiectasis rarely becomes apparent before the age of three years. Should it not be possible to control the symptoms with antibiotics and postural drainage, lung resection will be indicated.

The principles of physiotherapy are identical to those for adults. Extra care must be taken to maintain adequate humidification of the inspired gases and to prevent postural deformities. Detailed intensive treatment is described on page 87 *et seq.*

OPERATIONS ON THE PLEURAL CAVITY

Rarely is pleural disease primary; more often it is secondary to underlying disease. Pleural reaction may be dry, or associated with fluid collection due to altered osmotic pressures (transudates) (see page 180), or to inflammation (exudates). Causes of pleural exudates are:

   i) tuberculosis
  ii) neoplasm
 iii) pulmonary infarction
 iv) pneumonia
  v) subphrenic abscess
 vi) collagen disease.

Slow absorption of a large effusion may lead to fibrosis and subsequent lung restriction.

HAEMOTHORAX

This usually follows trauma to the chest wall which may in addition cause a pneumothorax, thus producing a haemopneumothorax. If the blood is not evacuated, organization, pleural fibrosis and lung restriction may occur.

EMPYEMA

This is a localized collection of pus in the pleural cavity, and may result from infection of pleural fluid or spread from a lung or subphrenic abscess. It may be the result of a wound infection and must be drained.

PNEUMOTHORAX

This is a collection of air in the pleural cavity, and may be: a) traumatic; b) spontaneous; c) therapeutic.

Traumatic pneumothorax. This may be caused by: i) trauma or surgical interference of the chest wall; ii) perforation of the trachea or oesophagus; iii) rupture of peripheral emphysematous cysts during coughing or artificial ventilation.

Spontaneous pneumothorax. This is caused by the rupture of a small vesicle on the surface of the lung (see page 184).

Therapeutic pneumothorax. Air may be introduced into the thorax to equalize intrathoracic pressures in a pneumonectomy space. The introduction of an artificial pneumothorax used to be a treatment for tuberculosis.

Operations performed on the pleural cavity are: pleurodesis; pleurectomy; decortication.

Pleurodesis

An artificial or chemical pleurisy is created by the introduction of an irritant to the pleural cavity. The ensuing pleural reaction results in the visceral and parietal pleurae becoming adherent, so preventing recurrent lung collapse.

Pleurectomy

This is performed through a standard thoracotomy incision and the parietal pleura is peeled from the chest wall. Any adhesions at the periphery of the diaphragm are freed. The visceral pleura will adhere to the chest wall, thus obliterating the pleural cavity.

Decortication

The thickened fibrotic restricting layer of visceral pleura is dissected off the lung surface. Thus the lung will expand fully and adhere to the parietal pleura.

Foreign matter and fluid are removed in pleurectomy and decortication. The chest is closed and drained with apical and basal intercostal tubes, until the lung is fully re-expanded. These tubes should never be clamped.

PRE-OPERATIVE PHYSIOTHERAPY

This follows the routine procedure. Specific instruction is given in diaphragmatic movement and unilateral costal movement.

POST-OPERATIVE PHYSIOTHERAPY

The immediate post-operative period is particularly painful and adequate analgesia must be given. The routine post-operative regime (described in Chapter 9) is instigated on the day of operation. Care of the drainage tubes, costal and diaphragmatic breathing exercises and coughing will be carried out with the patient in the side-lying position with the affected lung uppermost and the foot of the bed elevated. Efforts to regain maximum rib movement must never wane. The patient will sit out of bed on the first day and commence walking as soon as possible. All exercises are increased and postural drainage continued until intercostal tubes and/or all excess secretions are removed. Exercises in the ward class and gymnasium, and walking, must continue until discharge about the eleventh day. All movements should be unrestricted and the posture free and upright. Vital capacity and exercise tolerance should show improvement on the pre-operative assessment. If all parameters are not satisfactory the patient should attend for out-patient physiotherapy.

OPERATIONS ON THE CHEST WALL

Resection of whole or part of one or more ribs may have to be undertaken to excise a tumour. It may be necessary to repair extensive damage with a prosthesis. Sections of one or two ribs are resected to drain an empyema space. These wounds remain open for long periods, but may eventually be allowed to close.

Thoracoplasty

An extensive resection of ribs is undertaken and the chest wall, having no scaffolding, falls inwards and obliterates the pleural cavity and/or lung tissue. The operation used to be performed in cases of tuberculosis before suitable chemotherapy was instituted and lung resection became a common practice. Results of thoracoplasty may still be seen as the operation was performed up until the early 1950s. Infected pneumonectomy spaces or persistent bronchial stump fistulae are still closed in this manner. The first rib may or may not be removed.

Pre-operatively patients are often ill and weak following previous major surgery, illness or accident.

POST-OPERATIVE TREATMENT

This commences on the day of operation. Lateral costal and dia-phragmatic breathing exercises and coughing, full range active assisted shoulder movements and correction of position must be practised as soon as possible after the patient returns to the ward. The upper chest must be well supported during coughing, as there will be a paradoxical movement of the chest wall. The best position for the patient is forward sitting. The physiotherapist must hold the chest very firmly, with one hand on the back and the other over the upper part of the front of the chest.

First post-operative day. Bilateral and unilateral costal breathing exercises, diaphragmatic breathing exercises and coughing will be practised in side-lying, lying and half-lying positions. Leg, arm, shoulder girdle and head movements must be commenced. The patient will sit out of bed and walk around as soon as possible. Trunk exercises will begin on the second or third day. Intensive postural training is essential, especially in cases when the first rib has been resected.

Fractured Ribs

There will be surgical intervention only if the pleura and lungs are damaged. Pinning of multiple fractures is practised at some centres. The rib ends are approximated and fixed with medullary pins, thus reforming the rigid cage.

Major Injuries

Injuries of the chest wall occur frequently in road traffic accidents. Ribs may be dislocated or there may be numerous fractures. There is danger of the rib ends tearing the pleura and lung tissue. This results in bleeding and escape of air into tissues. A haemopneumothorax may ensue. The heart, mediastinum and great vessels are also at risk.

Multiple rib fractures result in a flail chest. Should a whole segment of ribs become detached *paradoxical breathing* will be present, which seriously compromises ventilation. On inspiration and expansion of the sound chest wall the intrathoracic pressure becomes negative and sucks *in* the disconnected portion of the chest wall. During expiration, as the sound ribs recoil, the increasing intrathoracic pressure pushes *out* the flail segment.

Not only does the flail segment move paradoxically, but so also does the air flow. As the flail chest is sucked in, air from the underlying lung is pushed into the unaffected side (should the injury be unilateral) resulting in adverse gas mixing.

TREATMENT

It is primarily necessary to maintain adequate ventilation. In massive injury an artificial airway is introduced and positive pressure ventilation established. Equal pressures are maintained intra-pulmonarily, thus adequately splinting the ribs and producing a symmetrical movement. Intermittent positive pressure ventilation via a tracheostomy may be necessary for up to three weeks or until the chest wall is stable. The treatment of the chest is described in the section on ventilators (see page 76 *et seq.*).

SPECIFIC TECHNIQUES FOR TREATING RIB FRACTURES

Excess secretions within the lung and pleural cavities must be evacuated. Pain and risk of further damage prevents any shaking manoeuvre at the site of injury. However, indirect vibration is particularly effective in these circumstances.

Methods

a) Institute shaking and percussion to the unaffected side during drainage of the affected side.

b) The shoulder girdle may be shaken down rhythmically onto

the chest wall by clasping both hands over the shoulder of the damaged side. This is particularly effective when the whole of the lower chest is involved.

c) Shakings over the actual area can be performed, if necessary, when the section is firmly splinted by a sustained high intrathoracic pressure. This situation occurs if the patient coughs whilst tracheal suction is in progress.

Congenital Deformities

PECTUS CARINATUM (PIGEON CHEST)
The sternum projects forward and is held in a prominent position by the ribs and costal cartilages.

Operation is undertaken to improve ventilatory capacity or (more commonly) for cosmetic reasons. The offending costal cartilages are removed and the sternum split horizontally and depressed. Fixation is established by suturing together both pectoralis major muscles in the mid-line.

PECTUS EXCAVATUM (FUNNEL CHEST)
The sternum is depressed in its lower end and with the in-turning costal cartilages forms a depression of varying degree. Ventilatory and cardiac function may be impaired and operation is performed to relieve this and for cosmetic purposes.

The costal cartilages are mobilized and the sternum split horizontally and may be held in its corrected position by a metal bar.

Post-operative physiotherapy follows the routine procedure for maintaining clear airways, lung expansion and preventing lung collapse. Shoulder girdle and arm exercises and postural correction are of particular importance.

Scoliosis and Kyphosis

Causes of scoliosis are: i) congenital; ii) idiopathic; iii) paralytic; iv) traumatic.

The reason for operation may be to correct deformity, to alter the growth potential, or for cosmetic purposes.

Operations which may be undertaken on the spine are posterior spinal fusion, multiple wedge resections, distraction or compression rods, or other compression forces on the convexity.

Cosmetic operations undertaken may be sub-total scapulectomy or costectomy.

Physiotherapy is of great importance to maintain adequate ventilation, increase muscle power and re-educate a good postural pattern. The vital capacity and the maximum voluntary ventilation (see page 40 *et seq.*) may be severely affected, as is the gas transfer and work of breathing. The patient will probably be nursed in a plaster bed or split plaster jacket for up to three months.

For references and bibliography, see end of Chapter 11.

Thoracic Surgery—III

by D. M. INNOCENTI, M.C.S.P.

CARDIAC SURGERY

INTRODUCTION

In 1938 Gross performed the first successful ligation of a persistent ductus arteriosus and opened the door to cardiac surgery. Modern techniques include closed and open procedures.

Closed heart surgery does not interfere with the circulation through the heart and the internal defect is corrected without direct vision. A small incision is made in the myocardium through which an instrument or finger is passed. Some external defects are repaired without interrupting the circulation.

Open heart surgery necessitates interfering with the circulation through the heart to obtain an unobstructed view of the lesion. The circulation and gaseous exchange is carried out by a heart-lung machine to maintain viability of all body tissues.

EXTRACORPOREAL CIRCULATION

Heart operations sometimes take a few hours. During this time the surgeon requires an empty and quiet heart. The process of blood circulation and oxygenation must be undertaken artificially. Venous blood is siphoned and gravity-drained from cannulae in the inferior and superior venae cavae or from the right atrium. The blood is oxygenated, cooled or heated, filtered and pumped back into a) the aorta (just above the aortic valve), or b) the femoral artery.

As the blood flow is taken onto bypass, the ventricular pressures fall and the heart stops pumping. At some centres the heart is made to fibrillate by an electric shock to prevent unwanted contractions. After the operation the heart may contract spontaneously as the intracardiac pressure increases with blood-flow. It may be necessary to promote the return to normal rhythm with a D.C. shock and local drug therapy.

The coronary arteries may remain unperfused without damage to the myocardium for up to 40 minutes at normal temperature, or longer with a hypothermic heart. It may be necessary to perfuse them with separate cannulae if the operation is prolonged.

OXYGENATORS

There are two types of oxygenators in general use and one under development.

Bubble oxygenators. Oxygen is bubbled into the bottom of an oxygenating tube, which contains the venous blood. The blood is arterialized as the oxygen bubbles rise. Excess gas is eliminated in the debubbling chamber and the blood filtered before entering the arterial line.

Disc oxygenators. A swiftly moving stream of blood is spread in a thin film onto discs (which may be stationary or rotating) and then exposed to an atmosphere of oxygen.

Membrane oxygenators. The natural process of oxygenation of blood occurs across a semipermeable membrane. In membrane oxygenators the blood film and the oxygen are separated by a stationary or rotating semipermeable membrane. Problems of size have not yet been overcome, and this machine is not yet in general use.

THE PUMPING MECHANISM

This must be capable of moving blood volumes of up to five litres/ minute against pressures of up to 180 mm Hg. The natural flow is pulsatile. The artificial flow is constant.

Filters are placed in the circuit to remove fibrin strands and debris.

Bubble traps are made of silicone-coated meshwork and are a necessary safety device to prevent air emboli from entering the circulation.

Heat exchangers maintain the normal physiological temperature against excessive heat loss in the circuit. They rapidly cool and re-warm the blood when necessary. As oxygen requirements are greatly reduced in cool tissues, difficult or long operations may be performed under hypothermia.

PRE-OPERATIVE PHYSIOTHERAPY

This follows the regime outlined on p. 193 *et seq*. It is particularly important to watch for signs of distress when positioning the patient. Many are unable to lie down due to heart failure. A knowledge of the drips, drains, leads and the possible need for ventilation is given to the patient. Those undergoing open heart surgery must know that the first few days will be spent in the intensive care unit.

POST-OPERATIVE PERIOD

Following a closed procedure, the patient will return directly to the ward. The regime is similar to the pulmonary scheme. The lung secretions will probably be less but general progress may be a little slower.

Following open heart surgery, the patient will return to the intensive care unit and may or may not be artificially ventilated. Continuous oxygen therapy will be in progress and in some cases Entonox will be administered. (Entonox is a mixture of nitrous oxide and oxygen which is used in the immediate post-operative hours for its analgesic and sedative effect.) The patient will be attached to:

a) an oscilloscope which shows the electrocardiograph;

b) venous lines for intravenous infusions, drug therapy and central venous pressure recordings;

c) an arterial line to which is attached a transducer or manometer which records the arterial pressure;

d) rectal and peripheral temperature probes;

e) urethral catheter;

f) Ryle's tube;

g) drainage tubes;

h) pacemaker leads.

Guide to Physiotherapy Progression Following Cardiopulmonary Bypass

Certain operative procedures and post-operative treatments are discussed in this section, but it must be emphasized that it is only possible to generalize. Each patient must always be assessed individually and at each treatment. Techniques must vary with the patient's condition and the surgeon's wishes.

217

Post-operative treatment and positioning is entirely dependent on the surgeon's wishes. Some do not wish their patients to commence physical treatment on the day of operation, nor to alter position for twenty-four hours. Others like to institute the first treatment as soon as the patient is co-operative, and allow alterations of position for physiotherapy and nursing procedures after the first few hours.

A. Treatment of Patients on Artificial Ventilation

Specific treatment of the chest during artificial ventilation and suction techniques are discussed in the section on intensive care (see Chapters 3 and 4).

B. Treatment of Patients Breathing Spontaneously

Special attention must be given to the cardiovascular state throughout the treatments.

DAY OF OPERATION

i) Breathing exercises and coughing. The patient is nursed flat or in half lying and general deep breathing must be encouraged by firm but gentle pressure of the physiotherapist's hands on the lower costal area. Huffing and coughing will be practised but it is rare for the patient to expectorate at this stage.

ii) Active plantar and dorsiflexion of feet.

iii) Passive or active-assisted knee flexion and extension, hip abduction and adduction approximately 6 to 10 times.

iv) Passive or active-assisted shoulder elevation and abduction approximately 6 to 10 times.

FIRST POST-OPERATIVE DAY

First treatment will be given as above and unilateral expansion exercises added. The physiotherapist supports the sternum with one hand, and gives gentle resistance with the other over the requisite area. Unilateral shakings over the lower and upper chest are also instituted to loosen secretions.

It will be necessary to support the incision and drainage sites during coughing.

Second treatment will be as for the first, but the patient should tolerate more breathing exercises, shakings and coughing.

Third treatment. All limb exercises should now be active-assisted or active. The patient may be turned for treatment, if his condition permits. The nurse in attendance will help to move and position the patient comfortably in side lying. Care of pressure areas and the change of bed linen will probably take place at these turning sessions.

The physiotherapist resists inspiratory efforts and assists expiratory efforts by manual pressure on the anterior and posterior aspects of the hemithorax under treatment. Shakings are given and huffing practised in this position. Adequate support must be given during coughing. If the patient's condition allows, the treatment is carried out on both sides.

The time spent in the side-lying position depends on the patient's cardiovascular and pulmonary condition. The latter is assessed by the daily morning X-ray and regular blood-gas measurements.

SECOND POST-OPERATIVE DAY

Transfer to the general ward may occur on the second or third day and depends on the condition of the patient's respiratory and cardiovascular systems. The physiotherapy is continued along previous lines. All limb exercises should now be active. Breathing, shaking and coughing exercises will continue in the lying and side-lying positions. It may be necessary to posturally drain a specific lung area and to add percussion over the back if sputum becomes particularly tenacious. Coughing may be more successful if the patient is supported in forward sitting.

THIRD, FOURTH AND FIFTH POST-OPERATIVE DAYS

Chest physiotherapy will continue two or three times a day, depending entirely on the X-ray appearances, blood-gas measurements, lung expansion and sputum production. It may be necessary to tip the bed for treatment if there are excess secretions, if the patient's condition allows.

Most surgeons like their patients to sit out of bed on the third or fourth day and start walking about on the fourth or fifth day. General arm and trunk exercises will now be done in the class.

Stair climbing may be commenced between the seventh and tenth days. About six stairs should be attempted the first time and the number increased over the next few days.

OPERATIONS

Heart operations will be considered in two sections:
A. Acquired lesions.
B. Congenital disorders.

A. ACQUIRED LESIONS

The Pericardium

Pericardectomy is performed to relieve the symptoms of chronic constrictive pericarditis. The pericardium is fibrotic and sometimes calcified due to previous tubercular infection. The constricted heart is unable to expand in diastole with resultant diminished cardiac output.

Incision: median sternotomy.

Closed procedure. The calcific and fibrotic pericardium is completely dissected and removed.

Post-operative physiotherapy. The routine post-operative treatment will commence on the day of the operation. Progress may be slow as exercise tolerance will be impaired due to the prolonged period of myocardial restriction. The patient will get out of bed about the third day and be discharged during the third week.

The Myocardium

Aneurysms may result from previous myocardial infarction. If high intracardiac pressures are maintained during the early post-infarction days there is risk of stretching the young fibrotic tissue. This ballooning of the wall of a cardiac chamber compromises the cardiac output and there is risk of rupture.

Infarcted tissue creates an akinetic area within the myocardium. If this is large the cardiac output is diminished. Cardiac failure may supervene.

Cardiomyopathy. In some myopathies the muscle may be greatly hypertrophied or the chambers enlarged. A forceful contraction becomes impossible, resulting in a diminished cardiac output.

Incision: median sternotomy.

Open procedure. Operations on the myocardium may involve: i) resection of aneurysm; ii) resection of infarcted tissue; iii) selective myocardial resection.

Pre- and post-operative physiotherapy. The treatment will follow the routine scheme, but progression will be slow as exercise tolerance is diminished due to protracted illness.

The Valves

The four valves lie in the same plane and one or more may become diseased causing them to become stenotic or incompetent (see page 268).

Operations on the valves are carried out under direct vision with a cardiopulmonary bypass, except for mitral valvotomy which is very successfully performed by a closed technique in certain circumstances. Valve surgery aims to repair or replace the deficient valve.

Valve Repair

CLOSED MITRAL VALVOTOMY
Incision: left thoracotomy through the fifth intercostal space.

Closed procedure. The heart is entered through the auricular appendage of the left atrium. The commissures of the valve are split with the finger, a small sharp instrument attached to the finger, or by special dilators. Rarely is this a permanent cure, but it affords good relief from symptoms. A further valvotomy or valve replacement may have to be undertaken in later life.

Pre- and post-operative physiotherapy follow the same routine as for thoracotomy. The progression of exercises may be a little slower than for lung resection. Discharge from hospital is on about the fourteenth day.

OPEN VALVOTOMY
This may be performed on the mitral, pulmonary or aortic valves. The commissures of the valves are split under direct vision with the patient on cardiopulmonary bypass. Aortic valvotomy carries a high risk of calcific emboli and is now rarely undertaken.

ANNULOPLASTY
This is a method of correcting a regurgitant valve by decreasing the size of the valve ring with sutures and securing Teflon.

VALVULOPLASTY
The cusps of a moderately involved valve may be sutured or re-

fashioned to produce an effective closure. In some selective instances repair or reconstitution of chordae tendinae is undertaken.

Incision: median sternotomy.

Pre- and post-operative physiotherapy will follow the routine cardiac scheme. After operation the patient is returned to the intensive care unit for the first 24 to 48 hours before transfer to the general ward. Discharge will be about the fourteenth day.

Valve Replacement

This is commonly undertaken as the treatment for incompetent or stenotic valvular lesions. Some valve prostheses available are:

a) *Starr-Edward.* A mechanical ball and cage device made of stainless steel. The early silicone ball type is being replaced by a steel ball type (see Fig. 11/1).

b) *Björk-Shiley.* A free-floating plastic disc suspended in a Stellite cage (see Fig. 11/1).

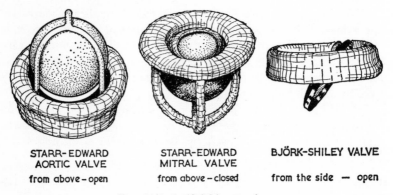

STARR- EDWARD
AORTIC VALVE
from above - open

STARR-EDWARD
MITRAL VALVE
from above – closed

BJÖRK-SHILEY VALVE
from the side — open

FIG. 11/1. Artificial heart valves

c) *Homograft.* A human valve may be dried, stored and reconstituted at the time of operation, or be treated with antibiotics and stored in a nutrient solution (see Fig. 11/2).

d) *Fascia lata graft.* A valve fashioned from the patient's own fascia lata. The majority of these valves have not survived the test of time.

Incision: median sternotomy.

Open procedure. The defective valve is excised completely and the prosthesis sutured securely into the valve annulus.

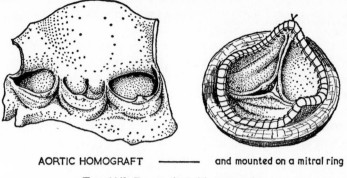

AORTIC HOMOGRAFT ———— and mounted on a mitral ring

FIG. 11/2. Reconstituted human valve

Pre- and post-operative physiotherapy will follow the routine by-pass scheme. Patients will be discharged, either to their home or to a convalescent home, after three weeks.

The Vessels

Grafts

Patients suffering from intractable angina or who have survived myocardial infarction may be found, by coronary angiography, to have operable occlusions of the coronary arterial system.

AORTOCORONARY ARTERY BYPASS GRAFT

This is perhaps the most recent advance in cardiac surgery, super-seding the Vineberg operation of implantation of the internal mammary artery into the myocardium (see References, page 242).

Incisions: median sternotomy and interrupted incisions along the course of the long saphenous vein.

The procedure is carried out under cardiopulmonary bypass. Part of the saphenous vein is removed and reversed to obliterate the valves. One end is anastomosed to the aorta, just above the aortic valve, the other anastomosed distal to the furthest block. Two or three grafts may be undertaken at one session.

Pre- and post-operative physiotherapy will follow the routine by-pass scheme. Discharge will be at about three weeks.

Thoracic Surgery—III

Resection and Anastomosis

Thoracic Aortic Aneurysms

Aneurysms of the aorta are results of trauma, hypertension, inflammation (syphilis), coarctation or atherosclerosis. They may be saccular or fusiform.

Dissecting aneurysm. Should the tunica intima rupture, the blood will flow between the intimal and medial arterial coats. The flow into connecting arteries will be compromised as the blood will bypass any arterial junction (see page 325).

Symptoms. An initial episode of acute pain is not always present. Symptoms are attributable to pressure on surrounding structures.

a) Venous engorgement from pressure on the superior vena cava, brachiocephalic vein or the right atrium.

b) Dyspnoea, cough or stridor from pressure on the trachea, bronchi or lung tissue.

c) Dysphagia caused by pressure on the oesophagus.

d) Alteration of speech and difficulty in coughing from pressure on the recurrent laryngeal nerve.

The roots of the innominate, subclavian and common carotid arteries may be occluded by clot or dissection. It is common for the aneurysm to rupture, fatally, into the pericardium, trachea or oesophagus.

Operation may not be indicated if there is massive distortion from syphilitic involvement.

Incision: is dependent on the site of the lesion, but usually it is a median sternotomy.

Procedure. The aneurysm is resected and the aortic ends anastomosed or reconstituted with a Dacron graft. If the vessels arising from the arch of the aorta are involved, they will be implanted into the graft. Repairs of aneurysms of the ascending aorta and aortic arch are carried out on cardiopulmonary bypass. Hypothermia is necessary if the cerebral circulation is affected. Venous blood is taken from the right atrium and returned to the femoral artery. Repairs of the descending aorta do not necessitate cardiopulmonary bypass.

Pre- and post-operative physiotherapy. Minimal pre-operative treatment is given to teach breathing exercises and the post-operative routine. There is great risk of rupture, so the patient is kept as quiet

224

as possible. Post-operative treatment will follow the routine by-pass scheme with discharge about the third week.

Pulmonary Embolectomy

Massive or repeated embolus may obstruct so much of the pulmonary vasculature that an adequate circulation cannot be maintained. Urgent operation may then be necessary.

Incision: median sternotomy.

Procedure. The operation is carried out on cardiopulmonary by-pass. The pulmonary artery is incised vertically and the embolus is lifted out. A sucker is passed into the right and left pulmonary arteries to ensure clearance of as many embolic fragments as possible.

It may be necessary to ligate the inferior vena cava to prevent further embolic incidents. This will be performed through a lateral *abdominal incision.*

Pre- and post-operative physiotherapy. The operation being an emergency procedure, there will be no pre-operative physiotherapy. Post-operative treatment will follow the routine bypass scheme.

Cardiac Myxoma

This is a rare condition of specific tumour formation within the cardiac chambers which most commonly arises in the left atrium. It is mobile and obstructs the mitral valve. The signs and symptoms are those of intermittent mitral valve disease. It may throw off emboli.

Incision: median sternotomy or left antero-lateral thoracotomy.

Open procedure. The heart is entered through the left atrium and the myxoma resected away from its root on the atrial wall. Alternatively, the right atrium is entered and the septum divided and removed with the pedicle and myxoma. The septum will be repaired or patched with Dacron.

Pre- and post-operative physiotherapy follow the routine bypass scheme. Discharge will be between ten days and three weeks.

Heart Block

This is a condition where there is interference in the normal conducting system of the heart. There are various degrees of the condition which may be due to:

i) Coronary artery disease.
ii) Myocarditis.
iii) Valve disease.
iv) Rheumatic fever.
v) Syphilitic heart disease.
vi) Diphtheria.
vii) Congenital disorder.
viii) Surgical interference.

In complete heart block the atria and ventricles work independently. The pulse rate is slow, usually between thirty and forty beats per minute. There is risk of attacks of unconsciousness during which the patient's pulse stops. Convulsions may occur if unconsciousness is prolonged. When the pulse returns the patient regains consciousness and may have a characteristic flush. Such periods of unconsciousness are termed *Stokes-Adams attacks*.

PACEMAKERS

An electrical device which artificially paces the heart is being increasingly used to correct the condition of heart block. There are two methods of inserting a permanent internal artificial pacemaker system, as follows:

1. Transvenous system. A cardiac catheter with a wire core and electrode tip is passed transvenously and embedded into the myocardium at the apex of the right ventricle. The pacemaker box is implanted subcutaneously in the axilla or epigastrium and connected to the electrode wire.

2. Epicardial system. Should the previous method be unsuccessful, it is necessary to perform a left thoracotomy and pericardotomy. Small electrodes are sutured to the epicardium and connected by screened wires to the pacemaker box, implanted subcutaneously as above.

A temporary pacing system may be necessary and will be fixed transvenously through the basilic vein or subclavian vein. The wires will be attached to an external pacemaker box.

Internal and external pacemaker systems may work on a fixed rate, on demand, or be atrial triggered.

Fixed rate pacemakers discharge at regular fixed intervals. The atrial and ventricular contractions will not be synchronized.

Demand pacemakers may operate in two ways. One type is linked to the interval between ventricular contractions. A ventricular contraction is sensed by the pacemaker, but should the next contraction be delayed the pacemaker will produce an impulse. The second type produces stimuli regularly. A spontaneous ventricular contraction will be sensed and the stimulus superimposed upon it (this will be ineffective as the myocardium will have depolarized). Should a ventricular contraction not take place the impulse will produce a contraction.

Atrial triggered pacemakers produce a near normal situation. An electrode situated in the right atrium relays the atrial impulse via a lead to the pacemaker box. The pacemaker then produces a stimulus which is relayed via a second wire and electrode to the right ventricle. As the atrial rate varies, so will the ventricular rate.

Post-operative physiotherapy. For transvenous implants—routine chest care with complete mobilization after twenty-four hours. For epicardial implants—routine post-thoracotomy scheme.

B. CONGENITAL DISORDERS

In order to help to understand these, a brief outline of the development of the heart is given here.

Development of the Heart

The heart is formed between the 21st and 40th days of embryonic life. Two symmetrically developing endothelial tubes fuse, commencing at the bulbar or arterial end, to form a tubular heart. As the tube grows in length, two grooves appear in the surface, which subdivide it into three primitive sections or chambers. The arterial end is called the *bulbus cordis,* the central chamber the *ventricle,* and the venous end the *sino-atrial chamber.* The groove between the ventricle and the sino-atrial chamber indicates the position of the *atrioventricular canal.*

The tube continues to increase in length. The middle portion grows more rapidly than the ends, resulting in the formation of a U-shaped loop, termed the bulboventricular loop (the right limb of the loop is formed by the bulb and the left limb by the ventricle).

The venous end of the tube (the common atrium) is pushed into an S-shaped curve and so lies above and behind the ventricular portion. A fold appears at the venous end of the atrium, dividing the chamber, to form the *sinus venosus.* Meanwhile, paired endothelial tubes arise to form the dorsal aortae, which grow down to the pericardium and join with the bulbus to form the *truncus arteriosus*.

The venous drainage is established by the union of an anterior cardinal vein from the head end of the embryo with a posterior cardinal vein from the tail end. This vessel then opens into the sino-atrial chamber by draining into the sinus venosus. The umbilical arteries and veins develop. These veins terminate in the sino-atrial chamber and will eventually drain into the right atrium.

The atria are formed from the common chamber.

The communication between the atrium and the ventricle (the atrio-ventricular canal) becomes divided by the formation of the atrio-ventricular endocardial cushions. These swellings grow from the centres of the ventral and dorsal walls of the canal, join together (thus forming the *septum intermedium of His*), and leave the right and left atrio-ventricular orifices, within which the mitral and tricuspid valves form.

The division between the right and left atria is formed by the growth of two septa.

The first septum, or *septum primum*, grows from the upper and dorsal part of the atrial wall down towards the endocardial cushions. It is necessary in the fetal heart for the two atria to communicate. The free passage of blood is maintained below the advancing edge of the septum. This communication is termed the *ostium primum*, and is low down, near to the atrio-ventricular canal. This hole decreases in size and finally closes as the septum encroaches on the endocardial cushions. To maintain an inter-atrial communication the dorsal part of the septum breaks down. This communication is termed the *ostium secundum* (foramen ovale) and is high up in the septum.

The second septum, or *septum secundum*, is formed by inflection of the muscular atrial wall, and it overlaps the septum primum at its periphery, leaving the centre free.

Whilst the septum is developing, a pulmonary vein opens into the left atrium and subsequently expands into the four pulmonary veins. The ventral walls of the atria bulge forwards, one on each side of the bulbus cordis, to form the atrial chambers.

The separation of the ventricles and of the truncus arteriosus into the aortic and pulmonary trunks are interrelated. Four endocardial cushions grow at the distal end of the bulbus (ventral, dorsal, right and left). The right and left cushions join to form the *distal bulbar septum*, which divides the orifice into ventral or pulmonary and dorsal or aortic sections. The four cushions eventually form the aortic and pulmonary valves.

Right and left spiral ridges appear within the truncus arteriosus and fuse together forming the *spiral aortopulmonary septum* (thus dividing the truncus arteriosus into the pulmonary trunk and the aorta). The proximal end of the septum fuses with the distal bulbar septum. The distal end of the aortopulmonary septum fuses with the aortic arches; thus one pair of arches fuse with the pulmonary trunk and the others with the aorta.

The separation of the ventricles occurs in three stages:

a) A muscular ridge projects into the ventricle to form the muscular septum, and fuses with the dorsal atrio-ventricular endocardial cushion, at its right extremity.

b) Right and left bulbar ridges fuse to form the *proximal bulbar septum*, and divide the bulbus cordis into pulmonary and aortic channels, which will continue up into the truncus arteriosus. The proximal bulbar septum fuses with the ventricular septum and the right extremity of the fused atrio-ventricular cushions.

c) The atrial septum fuses with the *centre* of the atrio-ventricular cushions and the ventricular septum with the *right extremity*. Hence, there is a portion of cushion dividing the right atrium from the left ventricle. It is this tissue which forms the membranous portion of the ventricular septum.

The mitral and tricuspid valves develop at the atrio-ventricular orifices by proliferation of endothelial tissue. *The aortic and pulmonary valves* develop from the four endocardial cushions at the distal end of the bulbus cordis.

The heart rotates to the left before birth and this rotation affects the final positions of the aorta, pulmonary trunk and valves, relative to each other.

Congenital disorders are considered in two groups:

ACYANOTIC GROUP
Cardiac disorders without associated shunting of blood or with shunting of arterial blood into the venous system (left to right shunt) do not produce a systemic cyanosis.

CYANOTIC GROUP
Conditions in which the pressure on the right side of the heart is

equal to or greater than that on the left, and have an abnormal communication between the two sides of the heart, allow venous blood to pass through the communication and mingle with the blood on the left. This reduces the oxygen content of the arterial blood and so produces systemic cyanosis.

The more common disorders may be listed as follows:

Acyanotic	*Cyanotic*
Coarctation of the aorta	Tetralogy of Fallot
Pulmonary stenosis	Transposition of the great vessels
Aortic stenosis	Pulmonary atresia
Persistent ductus arteriosus	Truncus arteriosus communis
Atrial septal defect	Tricuspid atresia
Ventricular septal defect	Anomalous pulmonary venous drainage

Corrective operations for most of the above conditions are open procedures on cardiopulmonary by-pass. The two exceptions are ligation of persistent ductus arteriosus and post-ductal coarctation of the aorta.

All conditions may be isolated lesions, or they may be combined with other defects. Each lesion will be considered separately in this text.

Coarctation of the Aorta

This is a constriction located at any site but most commonly just distal to the origin of the left subclavian artery (see Fig. 11/3). There will be an increased blood pressure proximal to, and a decreased blood flow distal to, the constriction. It may be due to contraction at the time of obliteration of the ductus arteriosus, or more possibly to embryonic malformation at the junction of the third, fourth and sixth aortic arches.

Symptoms. Patients may be asymptomatic or there may be headache, dizziness, tinnitus, epistaxis and palpitations due to increased blood pressure in the head and neck. Cold feet and possible claudication in the lower limbs are the result of decreased blood flow to the lower part of the body.

Incision: left postero-lateral thoracotomy through the fourth intercostal space.

Closed procedure. The coarctation is dissected and the ligamentum arteriosum or persistent ductus is ligated and divided.

230

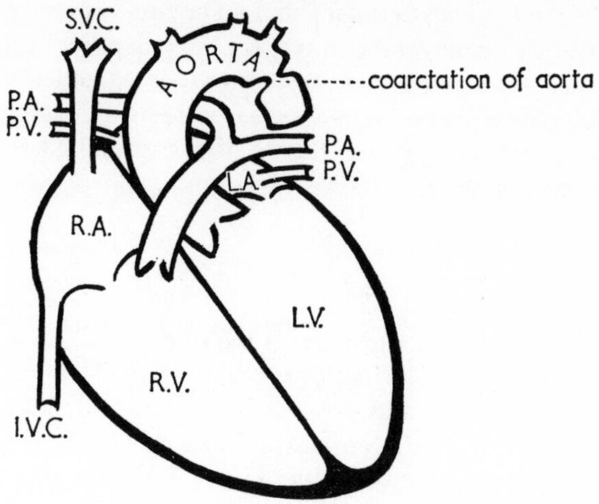

FIG. 11/3. Coarctation of the aorta

The divided ends of the aorta are anastomosed with Dacron sutures. Should the ends not approximate, a Dacron graft will be interposed.

Pre- and post-operative physiotherapy. Routine post-thoracotomy regime. The incision may extend very high posteriorly and special attention must be paid to posture and arm movements. Physiotherapy must not be vigorous. The blood pressure must not rise excessively, as it will put undue strain on the anastomosis site. Discharge is during the third week. Vigorous exercise should be avoided for a few months.

Pulmonary Stenosis

This is a congenital defect of fusion of the valve commissures, possibly in association with infundibular stenosis. The pulmonary circulation is decreased and the work of the right ventricle increased. This may result in right ventricular failure. It is probably due to failure of complete rotation of the left dorsal ridge during separation of the aorta and pulmonary artery.

Symptoms. Exertional dyspnoea, fatigue and possibly systemic venous congestion; hypoxaemia and cardiac failure in infants.

Incision: median sternotomy.

Open procedure. The valve is exposed via the anterior aspect of the pulmonary artery and the commissures are cut. If the annulus is constricted it is cut through vertically and a Dacron or pericardial gusset inserted. It may be necessary to replace the valve (see page 222).

Infundibular resection. The right ventricle is entered and the obstructing infundibular muscle and fibrosis is resected or the infundibulum is incised and a Dacron or pericardial gusset inserted.

Pre- and post-operative physiotherapy. Routine bypass scheme with discharge in the third week.

Aortic Stenosis

Left ventricular outflow obstruction may be caused at three levels, *a*) valvular, *b*) subvalvular, or *c*) supravalvular. This results in left ventricular hypertrophy and possibly left ventricular failure. It may be due to abnormal rotation of aortopulmonary septal ridges.

Symptoms. Mild—asymptomatic; severe—fatigue, syncope, effort dyspnoea and angina.

Incision: median sternotomy.

OPEN PROCEDURES

Valvular stenosis. Valvotomy is performed by entering the ascending aorta and incising the commissures.

Subvalvular stenosis. If the obstruction is due to a fibrous diaphragm arising from the ventricular septum, it may be approached through a low aortic incision and a through-valvular excision will be undertaken. When muscular sub-aortic stenosis is present, it may be corrected by selective myomectomy through a right or left ventricular incision.

Supravalvular stenosis. This is relieved by suturing an elliptical Dacron gusset into a vertical incision through the constricted portion of the aorta.

Pre- and post-operative physiotherapy. Routine bypass scheme with discharge in the third week.

Persistent Ductus Arteriosus

The ductus arteriosus, which connects the left pulmonary artery to the descending thoracic aorta just beyond the origin of the left subclavian artery, should have contracted, closed and fibrosed into the ligamentum arteriosum in a few days from birth. Occasionally it remains persistent and blood will flow from the aorta into the pulmonary system (see Fig. 11/4).

Symptoms. Asymptomatic or exertional dyspnoea. There is risk of subacute bacterial endocarditis and pulmonary hypertension.

Incision: left postero-lateral thoracotomy through the fourth intercostal space, or possibly a median sternotomy or submammary incision.

Closed procedure: ligation and dissection of ductus arteriosus under direct vision.

Pre- and post-operative physiotherapy. Routine thoracotomy scheme with discharge at about the eleventh day.

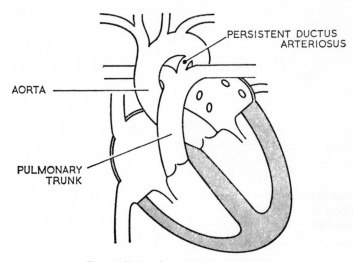

FIG. 11/4. Persistent ductus arteriosus

Atrial Septal Defect

Ostium secundum. This is a defect in the middle area of the septum. It is due to failure of fusion of the septum secundum to the septum primum to obliterate the foramen ovale. This is the most common and simplest to correct.

Ostium primum. The defect occurs low down in the septum and is sometimes associated with malformed mitral and tricuspid valves. It is due to defective formation of the interatrial septum as it fuses to the endocardial cushions. The operation is more complicated, because of the proximity of valves, coronary sinus, and the atrioventricular node.

233

Sinus venosus. This is a defect occurring high in the septum near to the orifice of the superior vena cava.

Symptoms. Secundum lesions may be asymptomatic or show mild exertional dyspnoea as the blood flows from the left to the right atrium, thus overloading the pulmonary system. Primum defects may produce extreme dyspnoea due to left ventricular failure if the mitral valve is involved.

Incision: anterior right thoracotomy through the right fourth inter-costal space, or a median sternotomy.

Open procedure. The heart is entered through the right atrium.

The secundum type is closed by direct suture. The primum type is repaired by insertion of a Dacron patch. If the mitral valve is involved it will be repaired first. Great care is taken to avoid damage to the atrio-ventricular bundle, which runs dangerously near to the operation site.

The sinus venosus type is sometimes associated with anomalous drainage of the pulmonary veins from the right upper lobe into the right atrium. The defect is repaired with a Dacron patch which re-directs the venous drainage into the left atrium.

Pre- and post-operative physiotherapy. Routine bypass scheme with discharge between ten days and three weeks.

Ventricular Septal Defect

This is perhaps the most common form of congenital heart disorder and involves the muscular or membranous portions of the septum. The defect may occur independently or be associated with other lesions. There are four common sites which are due to malformation of the ventricular septum, or to failure of fusion between the ventri-cular septum, the proximal bulbar septum and the atrio-ventricular endocardial cushions.

Blood is shunted through the defect from left to right, thus in-creasing the pulmonary blood flow and the return to the left atrium.

Symptoms. Patients with small defects may be asymptomatic. Large defects may cause exertional dyspnoea and right ventricular failure with systemic venous congestion.

Repair may be temporary in infants or complete after the age of three or four years.

TEMPORARY OPERATION

Relief is obtained by pulmonary artery banding (Muller & Dammann, 1952).

Incision: median sternotomy or left thoracotomy through the fourth intercostal space.

Closed procedure. The pulmonary artery is identified and its lumen restricted by a Teflon band. If the ductus arteriosus is persistent it is ligated and dissected.

REPAIR OF THE DEFECT

Incision: median sternotomy.

Open procedure. The heart is entered through the right ventricle. If the defect is small it can be repaired by primary suture. Larger defects are repaired with a Dacron patch.

Pre- and post-operative physiotherapy. Routine bypass scheme with discharge between eleven days and three weeks.

Tetralogy of Fallot

This is perhaps the most common form of congenital heart disease with cyanosis. There is (1) a high ventricular septal defect, (2) a pulmonary stenosis, which may be valvular, infundibular or a combination of the two, (3) an anomalous position of the aorta, and (4) hypertrophy of the right ventricle (see Fig. 11/5).

The anomaly results in a right to left interventricular shunt due to the right outflow tract obstruction and high right ventricular pressure. There is systemic cyanosis and risk of syncope. The child is usually undersized, has clubbing of fingers and toes, exertional dyspnoea and a spontaneous desire to squat. There is an acyanotic group of patients with the same anatomical abnormalities, but without severe pulmonary stenosis and therefore minor shunting.

The condition is probably due to the misalignment of the spiral ridges in the embryonic heart. This would account for the dextraposed aorta, small pulmonary trunk and abnormal valves and ventricular septal defect. The secondary hypertrophied right ventricle is due to outflow obstruction.

Correction may be palliative in the early years. Total correction is preferred between the ages of five and twenty-five years.

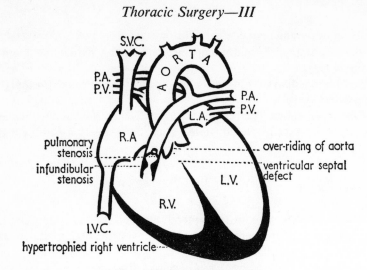

FIG. 11/5. Tetralogy of Fallot

ANASTOMOTIC PALLIATIVE TREATMENT

Waterston's anastomosis (ref.). Anastomosis of the ascending aorta and the right pulmonary artery.

Incision: right antero-lateral thoracotomy through the fourth intercostal space.

Potts' anastomosis (ref.). Anastomosis of the descending thoracic aorta to the left pulmonary artery.

Incision: left postero-lateral thoracotomy through the fourth intercostal space.

Blalock's anastomosis (ref.). Anastomosis of the pulmonary artery to the left subclavian artery.

Incision: left postero-lateral thoracotomy through the fourth intercostal space.

PALLIATIVE OR FIRST STAGE CORRECTION BY CLOSED PULMONARY VALVOTOMY

An expanding dilator (Brock ref.) or valvulotome is introduced into the outflow tract of the right ventricle and the pulmonary valve is dilated or cut.

TOTAL CORRECTION

Incision: this depends on previous palliative surgery. A left thoracotomy may be reused following a Potts' procedure. A median sternotomy or submammary incision will be used following a Waterston or Blalock procedure, and if there has been no previous intervention.

Open procedure. Existing anastomoses are closed prior to the intracardial total correction. The right ventricle is opened and a pulmonary valvotomy and/or infundibular resection carried out. The ventricular septal defect is repaired either by primary suture or by the insertion of a Dacron patch. The position of the Dacron patch will correct the position of the over-riding aorta.

Pre- and post-operative physiotherapy. Routine bypass scheme with discharge at about three weeks.

Complete Transposition of the Great Vessels

The aorta arises from the right ventricle and carries venous blood around the systemic system. The pulmonary artery arises from the left ventricle and carries oxygenated blood around the pulmonary system. In order for the patient to survive there must be communications between the two systems. Possible communications are persistent ductus arteriosus, atrial septal defect or ventricular septal defect (see Fig. 11/6).

In embryo the truncus arteriosus connects the ventricles to the

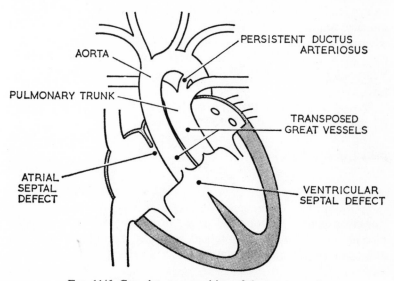

FIG. 11/6. Complete transposition of the great vessels

aortic arches. A septal division occurs and the truncal septum rotates through 225°. Should the rotation not be complete the great vessels will arise anomalously.

Symptoms. There may be cyanosis, syncope and dyspnoea.

PALLIATIVE OPERATIONS

Incision: right lateral thoracotomy through the fifth intercostal space.

a) The atrial septum is excised (Blalock & Hanlon, 1950), or ruptured (Rashkind & Miller, 1966), to create an atrial shunt.

b) The pulmonary artery may be banded to protect the pulmonary system from overloading, if there is a large ventricular septal defect (Sterns *et al*, 1965).

c) A side to side anastomosis of the aorta and pulmonary artery is undertaken if pulmonary stenosis restricts the pulmonary circulation.

CORRECTIVE OPERATIONS

1. Inflow tracts may be altered by transposing the pulmonary veins to the right atrium and the inferior vena cava into the left atrium. It may be necessary to use Dacron grafts (Baffes, 1956).

2. All inflow and outflow tracts may be retained but the venous return is redirected by excising the existing atrial septum and creating an artificial atrial septum fashioned from the pericardium. The pulmonary venous return in the left atrium is directed towards the tricuspid valve and right ventricle. The systemic venous return in the right atrium is entrained to the mitral valve and the left ventricle. Ventricular septal defects and anastomosis will be corrected (Mustard, 1964).

Pre- and post-operative physiotherapy. Routine post bypass scheme. Discharge is at about three weeks.

The following rare conditions are improved by reconstructive or palliative surgery:

Pulmonary Atresia

The pulmonary valve or trunk is malformed or deficient. The pulmonary blood flow is maintained by other communications, *e.g.* atrial and ventricular septal defects and a persistent ductus arteriosus.

Truncus Arteriosus Communis

A common pulmonary systemic trunk arises from the ventricles. There will be a ventricular septal defect and the trunk may or may not have two valves.

Tricuspid Atresia

The tricuspid valve is deficient and the right ventricle may be malformed. The pulmonary flow is maintained through atrial and ventricular septal defects and a persistent ductus arteriosus.

Anomalous Pulmonary Venous Drainage

All or some of the pulmonary veins may drain into the superior vena cava, the coronary sinus or directly into the right atrium. Sometimes the veins join behind the left atrium and are channelled into the brachiocephalic vein. Rarely drainage is into the inferior vena cava.

INFANTS

Infants and young children recovering from cardiac surgery are particularly prone to sudden and severe alterations in their condition, therefore meticulous estimations must be made concerning fluid balance, blood loss, blood sugar, and electrolytic and cardiac stability.

The heat-regulating centre in infants is unstable, so it is advisable to nurse them in a very warm, moist atmosphere. Immediately postoperatively babies may be nursed satisfactorily on a bed. An incubator has certain disadvantages, as it is difficult to manage the infant with drips and drains whilst maintaining adequate ventilation, humidification and oxygen concentrations. In some centres an infant nursing unit, with overhead heating, is found to be more convenient.

Ventilatory support is almost always necessary for 12 to 24 hours post-operatively. The correction of some congenital cardiac lesions will alter the pulmonary haemodynamics so drastically that ventilation may be needed for longer periods. Humidification must be such that the inspired gases are fully saturated.

Infants may need life-saving cardiac surgery in the first few weeks of life to relieve persistent heart failure and respiratory insufficiency.

The mortality risk is very high in the first few weeks of life, but lessens over the following months. The survival rate for infants over six months is high and comparable with that for older children.

Pulmonary complications are often the cause of death. Collapse and/or consolidation occurs rapidly in infant lungs: this necessitates frequent aspiration of the Jackson-Rees artificial airway (see Fig. 11/7). Suction in infants is a particularly delicate operation as it can precipitate the collapse of whole segments of lung. The suction catheter must be minute in calibre, and prolonged suction must be avoided. Should secretions be tenacious, the infiltration of 0·5 ml of saline to the trachea will promote aspiration.

The common congenital cardiac conditions have been previously described, but specific infant management will be mentioned.

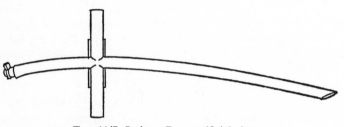

FIG. 11/7. Jackson-Rees artificial airway

COARCTATION OF THE AORTA

The majority of coarctations which have had to be surgically corrected in the neonate are pre-ductal. Re-coarctation may occur at the suture line, but this will be surgically corrected without difficulty when the child is older. The insertion of a graft is avoided for growth reasons.

PERSISTENT DUCTUS ARTERIOSUS

This is ligated in the neonate only if heart failure persists.

VENTRICULAR SEPTAL DEFECT

Only approximately one per cent of patients require surgery in the first few months of life. Pulmonary artery banding will be undertaken in infants under six months. Complete correction may be safely undertaken after the age of six months.

TETRALOGY OF FALLOT

Rarely is correction necessary in the first year of life. Should heart failure necessitate surgical intervention a shunt procedure will be undertaken.

TRANSPOSITION OF THE GREAT VESSELS

Palliative procedures undertaken within the first few months of life have improved the survival rate (up to three-quarters of those treated).

TOTAL ANOMALOUS PULMONARY VENOUS DRAINAGE

Severe heart failure appears very suddenly and an operative procedure will be undertaken as soon as a diagnosis is confirmed.

Pre- and Post-operative Physiotherapy

The principles of physiotherapy for children are similar to those for adults. Modifications are made in techniques, to allow for the size and frailty of the infant. If the child is conscious, limb movements are usually unnecessary. Full range passive movements will be carried out on the unconscious child.

Chest squeezing in time with the ventilator and shakings will be carried out by using the whole of the palmar surface of the fingers against the chest wall. An effective way of promoting a cough is to place the whole length of the fingers behind the chest bilaterally, mould the rest of the hands around the chest wall and shake the infant gently away from the bed. It will be necessary to position the child in side lying to drain and vibrate each lung separately. Should it be necessary to percuss the chest, it should be carried out with the fingers. Treatment will be necessary at least four-hourly during the period of artificial ventilation. It is beneficial to hyperventilate the lungs for a few breaths before re-settling the child onto the ventilator. This will ensure full expansion of lung tissue after suction.

Physiotherapy associated with bag squeezing may be undertaken. The techniques are as described in Chapter 4. An infant-sized bag will be used and precautions taken to allow for the frailty of the child. All manoeuvres must be performed with the palmar surfaces of the fingers, not with the whole hand.

When the cardiovascular and respiratory systems are stable, the child will move freely around the cot, and return home as soon as he is feeding and thriving.

REFERENCES

Baffes, T. G. (1956). 'A new method for surgical correction of transposition of the aorta and pulmonary artery.' *Surg. Gynec. Obst.*, **102**, 227.

Blalock, A. & Hanlon, C. R. (1950). 'The surgical treatment of complete transposition of the aorta and the pulmonary artery.' *Surg. Gynec. Obst.*, **90**, 1.

Blalock, A. & Taussig, H. B. (1945). 'The surgical treatment of malformations of the heart in which there is pulmonary stenosis or pulmonary atresia.' *J. Amer. Med. Ass.*, **128**, 189.

Brock, R. C. (1948). 'Pulmonary valvulotomy for the relief of congenital stenosis. Report of 3 cases.' *Brit. Med. J.*, **1**, 1121.

Muller, W. H. & Dammann, J. F. (1952). 'The treatment of certain congenital malformations of the heart by the creation of pulmonic stenosis to reduce pulmonary hypertension and excessive pulmonary flow. A preliminary report.' *Surg. Gynec. Obst.*, **95**, 213.

Mustard, W. T. (1964). 'Successful two-stage correction of transposition of the great vessels.' *Surgery*, **55**, 469.

Potts, W. J., Smith, S. & Gibson, S. (1946). 'Anastomosis of aorta to a pulmonary artery. Certain types in congenital heart disease.' *J. Amer. Med. Ass.*, **132**, 627.

Rashkind, W. & Miller, W. W. (1966). 'Creation of atrial septal defect without thoracotomy. A palliative approach to complete transposition of the great arteries.' *J. Amer. Med. Ass.*, **196**, 991.

Sterns, L. P., Ferlie, R. M. & Lilleheic, W. (1965). 'Cardiovascular surgery in infancy. Ten year results from the University of Minnesota Hospitals.' *Amer. Thoracic Surg.*, **1**, 519.

Vineberg, A. M. (1952). 'Treatment of coronary artery insufficiency by implantation of the internal mammary artery into the left ventricular myocardium.' *J. Thoracic Surg.*, **23**, 42.

Waterston, D. J. (1962). 'Treatment of Fallot's tetralogy in children under one year of age.' *Rozhl Chir.*, **41**, 181.

BIBLIOGRAPHY

Barnard, C. N. & Schrire, V. (1968). *The Surgery of the Common Congenital Cardiac Malformations*. Staples Press, London.

Brooks, D. K. (1967). *Resuscitation*. Edward Arnold, London.

Cleland, W., Goodwin, J., McDonald, L. & Ross, D. (1969). *Medical and Surgical Cardiology*. Blackwell Scientific Publications, Oxford and Edinburgh.

Clement, A. & Braimbridge, M. V. (1969). *Current Practice of Cardiopulmonary Bypass*. Blackwell Scientific Publications, Oxford and Edinburgh.

Emery, E. R. J., Yates, A. K. & Moorhead, P. J. (1973). *Principles of Intensive Care*. Unibooks, English Universities Press Ltd.

Gibbon, J. H. Jr., Sabiston, D. C. Jr. & Spencer, F. C. (eds) (1969). *Surgery of the Chest*. W. B. Saunders Co., Philadelphia, London and Toronto. 2nd ed.

Harris, E. M., Neutze, J. M., Seelye, E. R., Simpson, M. M. & Taylor, M. F. (1972). *Intensive Care of the Heart and Lungs*. Blackwell Scientific Publications, Oxford, London, Edinburgh and Melbourne.

Jones, R. S. & Owen-Thomas, J. B. (1971). *Care of the Critically Ill Child*. Edward Arnold, London.

CHAPTER 12

The Cardiovascular System, and Disturbances in Heart Rate and Rhythm

by E. A. BEAZLEY, M.C.S.P.,DIP.T.P.

The cardiovascular system consists of the heart and blood vessels.

The heart, a hollow muscular pump responsible for the circulation of the blood, is cone-shaped and lies in the thorax. Its base faces back up, and to the right, while its apex points down, forwards and to the left.

The atria form the base of the heart, the right atrium lying in front and to the right of the left. The apex is formed by the ventricles, the right ventricle forming a large part of the anterior surface of the heart.

Function of the Heart

The right side of the heart receives blood from the great veins and the coronary sinus, and transfers it to the pulmonary veins. The left side circulates the blood through the aorta to the body and its organs.

THE STRUCTURE OF THE HEART

There are four chambers in the heart: two atria and two ventricles separated longitudinally by an inter-atrial and an interventricular septum. The atria and ventricles are separated from each other by a circular fibrous septum or band.

The walls consist of three coats. An outer, the *pericardium*, is a containing and limiting membrane. It has two coats, an outer fibrous and an inner serous coat. The outer coat invaginates the heart and the roots of the great blood vessels. It is attached to the central tendon

243

of the diaphragm inferiorly, and is in close approximation with the parietal pleura of the lungs. The fibrous sac turns in on itself to form an inner serous lining which is in direct contact with the myocardium, and the fibrous outer layer.

The endocardium, the inner layer, lines the four chambers and forms the valves of the heart. It is formed of endothelial cells, which are continuous with the tunica intima of the blood vessels entering and leaving the heart.

The myocardium or muscular layer consists of superficial transverse and deeper longitudinal muscle fibres. The longitudinal fibres, which are arranged in a spiral manner, form the thicker layer; those forming the left ventricle, which pump blood through the systemic vascular system, are thicker than those forming the right ventricle. The atrial muscle fibres are about one-third of the thickness of the ventricular fibres.

The arrangement of cardiac muscle is known as a *syncytium* (Fig. 12/1). It is specialized muscle, striated in a longitudinal and transverse direction, and responds to the 'all or none' principle in its entirety. It has the inherent property of rhythmicity and starts to beat in an embryo before any nerve fibres have reached it.

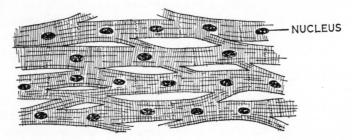

NUCLEUS

FIG. 12/1. Diagram illustrating the syncytial formation of cardiac muscle

The Valves

There are valves between the atria and the ventricles. The right has three cusps (tricuspid) and the left two (mitral or bicuspid) (Fig. 12/2). These valves are prevented from inverting by the chordae tendinae attached to the papillary muscles of the ventricular walls which act when the pressure in the ventricles is greater than that in the atria. A semilunar valve with three cusps lies between the right ventricle and the pulmonary artery, and another between the left

244

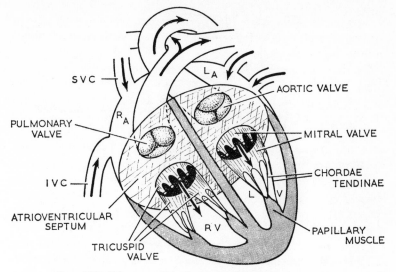

FIG. 12/2. Diagram of the heart showing its various valves

ventricle and the aorta. These open when the pressure inside the ventricles is greater than that in the blood vessels.

These four valves lie in the fibrous septum between the atria and the ventricles and on the same plane. They enable the ventricles to pump blood through the body effectively. Any abnormality leads to the heart becoming inefficient as a pump (see Fig. 12/3).

The Surface Marking of the Heart

The apex lies in the fifth intercostal space, 9 cm from midline. A convex line drawn up to the left second costal cartilage at its junction with the sternum, passing across to the right third costal cartilage 2·5 cm from the sternum, and down to the right sixth costosternal junction, and then concave to the apex, will outline the heart (Fig. 12/4).

The Conducting Mechanism

This consists of specialized muscle and nerve fibres which super-impose a faster rate of contraction on the normal heart muscle and transmit this contraction wave from the atria to the ventricles.

245

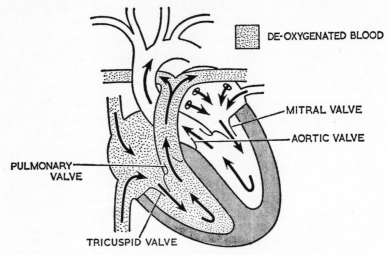

FIG. 12/3. Diagram showing the blood circulating through the valves

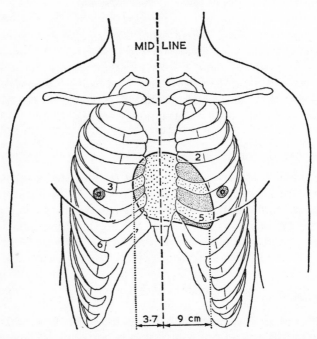

FIG. 12/4. Anterior aspect of the thorax showing the surface projection
of the heart

The sino-atrial node lies in the right atrium close to the junction of the great veins. It is a small mass of specialized muscle and nerve fibres embedded in connective tissue. The normal rhythmicity of this tissue is higher than that of cardiac muscle, and is the rate at which the whole of the heart contracts under normal conditions. It is often termed the 'pacemaker'.

The atrioventricular node lies in the distal part of the inter-atrial septum close to the coronary sinus. It is formed of specialized muscle fibres, nerve cells and fibres.

The atrioventricular bundle passes from the atrioventricular node across the atrioventricular septum and divides into right and left limbs. These pass down in the ventricular muscle lying on either side of the interventricular septum. On reaching the apex they turn in towards the papillary muscles and divide into plexi. The branches spread out through the ventricular myocardium and are known as Purkinje fibres.

THE HEARTBEAT

Cardiac muscle has the property of rhythmicity and will contract and relax on its own, producing a beat which is associated with electrical changes of depolarization and repolarization. This ability is developed to its maximum at the sino-atrial node near the orifice of the superior vena cava. In a fully developed heart each heartbeat originates at the *sino-atrial node*. The contraction waves spread from the pacemaker through both atria, causing them to contract simultaneously and force blood, which is in the atria, through the atrioventricular valves into the ventricles. Blood is prevented from regurgitating into the great veins by closure of the rings of cardiac muscle round the orifices during the contraction.

The electrical charges do not take place across the fibrous atrioventricular septum, but are conducted from the muscular atria to the *atrioventricular node* sited near the atrioventricular junction of the right atrium. They then pass down the atrioventricular bundle (bundle of His) lying in the anterior interventricular septum to enter the ventricular muscle near the apex. The conduction waves spread up towards the base, forcing the blood towards the aortic and pulmonary valves (Fig. 12/5).

Bundle branch block occurs if there is disease of the myocardium interfering with the transmission down one limb of the atrioventricular bundle.

247

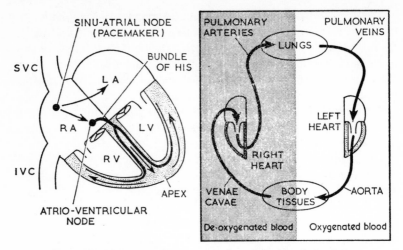

Fig. 12/5. Diagrammatic representation of the blood circulation

Heart block occurs when the atrioventricular bundle is damaged. The conduction wave is interrupted and does not reach the apex of the ventricles, and so the ventricles beat at their slower inherent rate, independent of the atria.

Blood Supply of the Heart

The heart is supplied by two coronary arteries arising from the ascending aorta directly above the aortic valve. They are filled when the heart muscle is relaxed (diastole). Except at their most proximal part they anastomose freely and form a vast capillary network throughout the myocardium (Fig. 12/6).

The right coronary artery from the anterior aortic sinus supplies the right atrium and both ventricles posteriorly. A branch supplies the sino-atrial and atrioventricular nodes and the main atrioventricular bundle. The limbs of the bundle are supplied by both right and left coronary arteries.

The left coronary artery from the left posterior aortic sinus supplies the left atrium and both ventricles anteriorly.

The endocardium and valves have no blood supply.

The majority of the veins of the heart drain into the right atrium at the coronary sinus. The remaining small vessels drain through the walls of the heart into the right or left atrium.

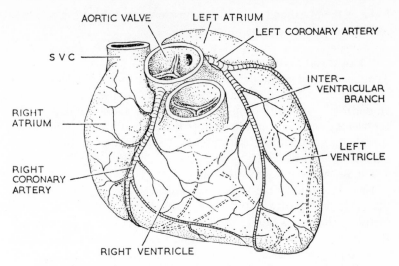

FIG. 12/6. Anterior aspect of the heart showing the coronary vessels

The Nerve Supply to the Heart

The autonomic nervous system supplies the heart with a *sympathetic* and a *parasympathetic* supply. It is thought that these interact under normal conditions, so that if there is decreased vagal (parasympathetic) activity leading to an increased heart rate, there will be an increased sympathetic activity at the same time.

The cardiac centre which controls sympathetic and vagal tone lies in the medulla, and is in turn subject to a higher control from the cortex and hypothalamus.

THE SYMPATHETIC SUPPLY

Nerve cells lie in the upper five thoracic segments of the lateral horns of the spinal cord. Axons pass from these segments to the superior, middle, and inferior cervical ganglia, synapse and pass to the heart via the superior, middle and inferior cardiac sympathetic nerves. These nerves supply the sino-atrial node, atrioventricular node, and the atrial and ventricular muscle. The chemical transmitter at these postganglionic nerve endings is *noradrenaline.*

The sympathetic system is stimulated at times of stress, *e.g.* fright, or during haemorrhage. This leads to an increased heart rate and speed of conduction of the heartbeat, and an increased contraction

249

force of the atrial and ventricular muscle so that there is a maximal increase in the cardiac pumping action.

THE PARASYMPATHETIC SUPPLY

The vagal nerve cell bodies lie in the dorsal motor nucleus of the vagus in the medulla. Preganglionic fibres travel in the vagi (tenth cranial) synapsing with ganglion cells near the sino-atrial node, atrioventricular node and in the wall of the atria. Postganglionic fibres supply these structures. The chemical transmitter at these nerve endings is *acetylcholine*.

The ventricles have no vagal supply.

The vagi monitor the sino-atrial node, the natural rhythmicity of the node being higher than the normal heart rate. Vagal tone (activity) slows this rate to the normal (about 75 beats per minute). If vagal tone increases, the heart rate becomes slower, *e.g.* during sleep; on waking the vagal tone decreases and the heartbeat quickens.

THE CARDIAC CYCLE

This is the sequence of events which takes place on an average of 70 times per minute in inactivity (resting heart rate).

The heart muscle is in a state of contraction, systole, or relaxation, diastole, throughout.

The cycle is 0·8 seconds long and is made up of an atrial part (systole 0·1 seconds and diastole 0·7 seconds), and a ventricular part (systole 0·3 seconds and diastole 0·5 seconds). This gives a complete diastole (atrial and ventricular) of 0·4 seconds (Fig. 12/7).

The events start while the atria are relaxed and filling with blood from the great veins. Isometric ventricular diastole begins, atrial pressure rises and the atrioventricular valves open, allowing blood to flow rapidly and then more slowly through to the ventricles. The pressures become almost even in the atria and ventricles; after 0·4 seconds of ventricular diastole the heartbeat is initiated at the sino-atrial node and a contraction wave spreads over the atria, the great veins are sealed and pressure increases in the atria and ventricles. This pressure reduces as the wave diminishes and is transmitted by the atrioventricular node and bundle to the apex of the ventricles; as the contraction enters the ventricles the interventricular pressure rises and the atrioventricular valves float up and shut (first heart sound LUBB) and are prevented from inverting by the

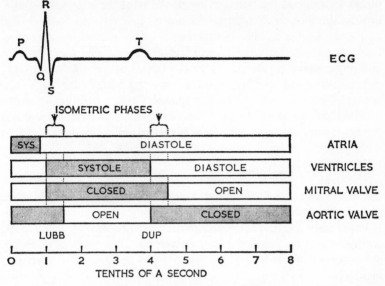

FIG. 12/7. Diagrammatic representation of the cardiac cycle

tension of the chordae tendinae. There is an isometric contraction of the ventricles causing the pressures in the enclosed ventricles to rise rapidly, exceeding that in the aorta and pulmonary artery, opening the semilunar valves and ejecting blood into the arteries. As blood is ejected, pressure increases in the blood vessels and decreases in the ventricles; the valves snap shut (second heart sound DUP) and the ventricles begin to relax, and the cycle is repeated.

Cardiac Output

This is the quantity of blood pumped out by each ventricle per minute. It depends on the heart rate and the stroke volume and may be expressed thus:

Cardiac output = heart rate (1) × stroke volume (2).

1. The heart rate is the number of cardiac cycles per minute (see cardiac cycle).

2. The stroke volume is the amount of blood pumped out by each ventricle per beat. This is determined by the amount of blood in each ventricle at the beginning of ventricular systole. The quantity of

251

blood depends on the size and distensibility of the ventricles in relation to the quantity contained in the venous system (systemic and pulmonary), which is about three-fifths of the circulating blood.

If the thin-walled veins contract, decreasing their total capacity, and more blood is forced into the ventricles, there will be a greater volume of blood and more stretch on the ventricular wall. The ventricle will respond by contracting more forcefully (Starling's law).

Starling's law of the heart ensures that the right and left sides of the heart have an equal output of blood per minute.

Control of the Heart Rate

The heart rate depends on the rate at which the sino-atrial node initiates the heartbeat.

Vagal tone (*activity*) originates in the cardiac centre of the medulla, and decreases the heart rate by its action on the sino-atrial node (see nerve supply of the heart). If vagal activity decreases the heart rate increases.

Stimulation of the *sympathetic nervous system* (flight or fright mechanism) results in an increased heart rate and an increased force of contraction by the ventricles. The chemical transmitter is noradrenaline.

Baroreceptors which maintain the blood pressure at a constant level record the degree of stretch on the walls of the carotid sinus, the subclavian artery and the arch of the aorta. If the blood pressure rises, increasing the stretch on these arterial walls, the baroreceptors cause the cardiac centre to slow the heart rate. Should blood pressure fall, decreasing the stretch on the arterial wall, the cardiac centre will stimulate the heart to beat quicker, *e.g.* haemorrhage.

Chemoreceptors which respond to an alteration in the blood gases primarily affect the respiratory system.

Respiration. During quiet respiration in a normal adult the heart remains constant, but on deep breathing the heart rate increases during inspiration, but slows during expiration. This alteration in rhythm is known as *sinus arrhythmia.*

There is a *higher centre of control* than the medulla in man. This is probably responsible for the increased heart rate under *emotional stress, e.g.* prior to public speaking, or before a competition. It has been demonstrated that the heart rate can be increased to 200 beats per minute in some circumstances of stress.

The adrenal medulla secretes two hormones, noradrenaline and adrenaline, which have a direct effect on the heart, and increase its rate at time of *emotional excitement*.

Temperature changes have a direct effect on the heart rate. Lowering of the body temperature (hypothermia) decreases the heart rate, and an increase in heart rate occurs with an increased body temperature, *e.g.* a fever (normal 37° C), a hot bath, or sunbathing extensively.

Thyroxine liberated from the thyroid gland stimulates the sino-atrial node to beat faster. If there is an increase in the normal quantity of circulating thyroxine, *e.g.* in thyrotoxicosis, the patient will have a fast heart rate.

Pain is conducted by the sensory nerves and slight pain is associated with an increased heart rate, but with severe pain there may be a decreased heart rate.

All active and passive movements will affect the cardiac output and the factors affecting them are included above.

DISTURBANCES OF CARDIAC RATE AND RHYTHM

Disturbances of cardiac rate and rhythm are due to disturbances in forming electrical impulses or to failure to conduct these impulses correctly.

IMPULSE FORMATION

The normal heart rate varies but has an average rate of 70 rhythmical cycles per minute at rest. The electrical impulse is initiated at the sino-atrial node (pacemaker) and spreads out over the atria; it is picked up by the atrioventricular node and conducted by the atrioventricular bundle to the apex of the ventricles.

FACTORS INFLUENCING IMPULSE FORMATION

The rhythmical contraction of the myocardium is under the control of the autonomic nervous system, and may be affected by vagal tone (inhibitory), sympathetic impulses (excitatory); indirectly by emotion, directly or indirectly by chemicals, *e.g.* noradrenaline, thyroxine; by body temperature changes and indirectly by pain.

The sino-atrial node receives its blood supply from a branch of the right coronary artery. Coronary vascular disease could impair the nutrition of the pacemaker which would interfere with the node's function.

IMPULSE DISORDERS

Impulses initiated at a faster rate than normal are known as *sinus tachycardia*, at a slower rate *sinus bradycardia* and of an arrhythmical type are known as *sinus arrhythmia*.

Occasionally other areas of the heart begin to initiate impulses. These are known as *ectopic foci* and can occur in either atria or ventricles. These foci produce premature beats which interrupt the normal heart rhythm. If listening to the heart, the next normal beat may not be heard as the muscle will still be in the refractory state.

Important alterations in rhythm resulting from ectopic foci are both atrial and ventricular tachycardias, an atrial flutter, and atrial and ventricular fibrillation.

Atrial or Ventricular Tachycardia

This is nearly always paroxysmal and consists of a succession of rapid rhythmical premature beats. The attacks usually pass off suddenly. In each case there may be no underlying heart disease but anoxia of the ventricular muscle, or an overdose of digitalis, may be the cause of ventricular tachycardia, *e.g.* following myocardial infarction. The attack is accompanied by palpitations, anxiety and weakness.

TREATMENT

D.C. electroversion may be used in both instances to re-establish a normal rhythm (see ventricular fibrillation).

Atrial tachycardia may be treated by drugs, *e.g.* digitalis, providing this has not been the cause of the tachycardia.

Ventricular tachycardia may be treated by a myocardial depressant such as propranolol to try to re-establish normal rhythm.

Atrial Flutter

Atrial flutter is due to a rapid regular stimulus formation in an ectopic form producing contraction waves at the rate of about 300 per minute. The functional tissue is unable to respond at this rate, due to the natural refractoriness of the atrioventricular conducting tissue, and will induce ventricular contractions at a rate of 2:1, 3:1 or 4:1 (partial atrioventricular block). If this rate continues for some days or longer, congestive failure is likely to develop.

Atrial Fibrillation

This differs from atrial flutter in its speed. The stimulus formation is more rapid (450 per minute or more), and irregular. The atria appear to be 'twitching' rather than contracting and they no longer eject blood into the ventricles. The danger of this is the possible formation of clots in the atria, particularly in the left auricular appendage. Clots may be dislodged from the left side causing cerebral or systemic arterial emboli, or from the right side causing pulmonary emboli.

The effect on the ventricles depends on how many contraction waves spread to the ventricles. If a high proportion reach the ventricles cardiac failure is likely to ensue.

In both atrial flutter and fibrillation there is usually underlying heart disease, which is most commonly mitral stenosis.

The object of treatment is to restore sinus rhythm, and lower the rate of conductivity so that fewer stimuli reach the ventricles. This can usually be achieved by the use of digitalis.

Ventricular Fibrillation

This type of fibrillation is characterized by rapid irregular ineffectual twitchings of the ventricles. They do not produce an adequate cardiac output, and so this condition is likely to be rapidly fatal. It is usually the cause of death following coronary thrombosis. Sometimes it can be arrested by the use of the defibrillating machine. In this method an electric shock depolarizes the myocardium and when the heart begins to beat again it is hoped that the normal rhythm will be re-established.

Interference in Conduction

This is known as *heart-block*. The interference may be in any part of the conducting system, but the commonest sites are the atrioventricular node and the atrioventricular bundle. The lesion is usually calcification or fibrosis of the conducting system which occurs in coronary artery disease or chronic rheumatic carditis; or it may be a congenital defect.

The passage of the impulse is either delayed (partial heart-block) or prevented (complete heart-block). The atria and ventricles beat independently and if no impulse reaches the ventricles they beat at their inherent rate of about 40 per minute. This ventricular rate cannot change to meet the varying needs of the body.

The danger of this condition is the occurrence of *Stokes-Adams attacks* which may prove fatal. Occasionally in heart-block the slow ventricular rate changes to ventricular tachycardia or fibrillation; or as a partial heart-block changes to a complete heart-block the ventricles stop; in each case the patient becomes unconscious and pulseless. Convulsions develop due to cerebral anoxia, breathing becomes stertorous and the sufferer becomes deeply cyanosed. After about half a minute the ventricle starts to beat again, which may be due to anoxia; convulsions cease and the patient's colour and pulse return.

TREATMENT

Treatment of acquired heart-block is usually by the administration of drugs which quicken the heart rate, but if these are ineffective and there are frequent Stokes-Adams attacks the rate of ventricular contraction may be controlled by an artificial pacemaker (see page 226).

For references and bibliography, see end of Chapter 16.

CHAPTER 13

Cardiac Failure

by E. A. BEAZLEY, M.C.S.P., DIP.T.P.

The heart, a muscular pump, supplies the metabolic needs of the tissues. The needs vary, the tissues demanding more on exercise and less at total rest. They are met by a rapid response which alters the force, or the rate of contraction of the heart, or both.

The heart responds like voluntary muscle, and can increase its output on severe exertion; or if necessary, providing there is an adequate oxygen supply to the myocardium, it will hypertrophy, as for example in athletes.

The cardiac reserve and ability to hypertrophy enable the myocardium to cope with damage or disease, *i.e.* to compensate, so that an individual may have a heart lesion for years but be totally unaware of it.

When the oxygen supply becomes inadequate for the increased needs of the now hypertrophied myocardium, the heart muscle ceases to hypertrophy and the strength of contraction gradually fails to maintain an adequate output. The cavity dilates and back pressure causes a rise in venous pressure. Signs and symptoms of heart involvement appear and the heart is said to be decompensating or failing.

Compensation is the ability of the myocardium to respond to more work, by hypertrophy. The area of hypertrophy depends on the site of the lesion. At first there will be an increased volume of blood in a chamber, *e.g.* the left ventricle with aortic stenosis. The ventricle dilates slightly, which stimulates a stronger contraction to overcome the resistance and maintain a normal output volume. This will occur over a long period but eventually the limit of hypertrophy will be reached. *Decompensation* then follows. Output begins to fall and the

257

ventricle dilates. This decompensation is made more likely as the nutrition of the subendocardial muscle is impaired by the high ventricular pressure, and ischaemic fibrosis gradually develops.

There are no symptoms of impending failure while the heart's chambers are responding by hypertrophy. As compensation fails, symptoms appear on severe exertion, so that the patient decreases his activity. Fatigue and breathlessness gradually appear on mild exercise such as walking, and eventually symptoms appear at rest. This is *cardiac failure*.

The whole heart, all four chambers, may fail together, but frequently the clinical picture is one of failure of one side more than the other.

Left ventricular failure usually occurs in association with hypertension when the peripheral resistance is high. Disease of the aortic valve, either stenosis or incompetence, or both together, force the left ventricle to work harder, to hypertrophy and eventually to fail. Coronary artery disease and myocardial infarction may cause left ventricular failure. The disease of the coronary vessels deprives the heart muscle of adequate oxygen, and ischaemic fibrosis develops.

Left atrial failure occurs where there is an obstruction to the flow of blood into the left ventricle as in mitral stenosis, and there is a reservoir of blood left in the atrium following each phase of emptying.

Left-sided heart failure is the failure to maintain an adequate circulation of the systemic flow of blood, and so the needs of the tissues are not met, and the patient feels weak and lethargic.

Right ventricular failure may follow left ventricular failure, as there is back pressure exerted through the pulmonary circulation to the right ventricle. When the pulmonary hypertension becomes too great, the right ventricle fails.

Pulmonary hypertension leading to right ventricular failure will occur in the presence of emphysema or any other disease of the lung, which reduces the capillary field. Disease of the pulmonary arteries, *e.g.* pulmonary embolus, restricts the circulation of the blood to some extent, causing the right ventricle to work harder and eventually fail.

Congenital heart disease, *e.g.* septal defects, or stenosis of the pulmonary valve, and any condition which interferes with the return of blood to the heart or to the right ventricle, *e.g.* tricuspid valvular disease, will result in right-sided failure.

Right-sided failure, where there is an inadequate return of blood from the periphery to the heart, results in peripheral oedema often seen in the feet and sacral areas, and in the enlargement of the liver.

Heart failure will occur in the presence of *thyrotoxicosis* when too many demands are made on the heart. However thyrotoxicosis is usually a precipitating factor, not a cause of heart failure.

Congestive Cardiac Failure

This is a term which is usually applied when the left side of the heart fails and the lungs become congested. Ultimately there is congestion of the peripheral circulation, but this may not be in evidence at first.

The congestion may be in the pulmonary system, or in the systemic system, or in both systems. It is usually due eventually to the retention of sodium and water by the kidneys resulting in a larger blood volume.

In left-sided congestive failure the left side of the heart fails to provide an adequate pump and pulmonary congestion develops. The pulmonary vessels constrict, increasing the work of the right ventricle. While the right side of the heart continues to pump adequately, pulmonary congestion gradually increases. There will be oedema of the lung parenchyma and, as it increases and becomes chronic, there is thickening of the interstitial tissue and the lungs become 'stiff'. It is harder to expand them and the free interchange of gases is reduced. Breathing difficulties gradually increase.

Dyspnoea (difficulty with breathing) is the outstanding feature. It occurs on exertion at first and gradually at rest. Orthopnoea and paroxysmal nocturnal dyspnoea gradually appear.

Congestion of the pulmonary system increases with exercise. The lungs become stiffer and more waterlogged. The chronic oedema causes interstitial thickening and more force is required to expand the lungs. Breathing becomes shallow and the respiratory rate increases. Any increase in venous return increases the pulmonary congestion.

Orthopnoea—discomfort in the lying position—occurs because there is an accumulation of blood in the lungs in lying.

Paroxysmal nocturnal dyspnoea occurs during sleep. The patient slips down in bed and congestion occurs. During sleep the respiratory centre is less responsive, the PCO_2 rises and the patient wakes to a a feeling of suffocation, sits on the side of the bed or walks to a window. The upright position relieves the congestion and the 'attack' passes off. In advanced failure relief is slow, acute pulmonary oedema develops and, if the attack of 'cardiac asthma' passes, it is followed by an unpleasant cough with copious frothy white or blood-stained sputum. An acute attack may be fatal.

The complications of left-sided failure are chest infection, deep venous thrombosis and pressure sores. The latter may occur because the patient is nursed in sitting and may not be able to turn very far from one side to another.

There will be general muscular weakness and there may be a lack of tone in the interossei and lumbricals of the feet. If the bed-clothes have been too tight and the feet not fully dorsiflexed with the knees straight, the tendo achilles may shorten slightly.

In right-sided congestive failure the signs and symptoms of systemic venous congestion, due to an inadequate pumping action on the right side, are visible. These are pulsation of the veins at the root of the neck above the medial third of the clavicle; distention of the external jugular vein; a swollen tender liver palpable below the costal margin which may cause pain sited in the right hypochondrium, due to stretching of the liver's capsule; loss of appetite and nausea with vomiting because of the portal congestion; ascites if there is an outpouring of serous fluid into the peritoneal cavity; oedema of the periphery and cyanosis.

Oedema of cardiac failure usually has a low protein content as it is due to high veno-capillary pressure. The fluid gravitates and is seen in the most dependent parts, feet and ankles when the patient is up, and the sacral region when the patient is recumbent. It may be detected by applying pressure over the area with the pad of the thumb for one or two seconds. On release the impression of the thumb will remain for a short while (pitting oedema).

Peripheral cyanosis will occur if the right-sided failure is secondary to left-sided failure, but it is not very marked. It occurs because there is a poor peripheral circulation with slowing of blood in the capillaries, giving more time for diffusion of gases. It disappears if the extremities are warmed.

Central cyanosis occurs if there is disease of lungs causing deficient oxygenation of blood. It is not relieved by warming.

In right and left heart failure there are changes in the electrocardiogram, in the PCO_2 and PO_2 levels, in the normal X-ray picture, and in the heart sounds.

COMPLICATIONS OF CONGESTIVE CARDIAC FAILURE

Patients are prone to chest infections. Pressure sores tend to occur because patients may be on bed rest for a long period, and oedema and lack of nutrition to the tissues makes them particularly susceptible to pressure sores.

Renal failure may be a complication if there is damage to the kidneys and if the fluid restriction is too great.

TREATMENT OF CARDIAC FAILURE

The main principles of treatment are to remove or alleviate the cause of failure; to reduce the demands on the heart during failure; to improve the function of the myocardium; to reduce the extracellular fluid and plasma volume.

Removal of the cause may be possible if it is a mechanical defect which can be treated by surgery. However, surgery is usually delayed until the myocardium is in as healthy a state as possible. Hypertension is relieved by anti-hypertensive drugs. Lung infections will be treated with antibiotics and physiotherapy. Urinary obstruction must be relieved, and recurrent rheumatic fever or subacute bacterial endocarditis will be treated by drug therapy, usually penicillin.

Reducing the demands on the myocardium requires rest in an armchair, a cardiac bed with the legs dependent or in half lying and relief of fear and anxiety, with adequate sleep. Rest will vary in length of time, but is usually for a period of about three weeks, or until the oedema has reduced. Relaxation may need to be taught to very tense patients to improve their ability to rest. The conscious method would be used so that no extra work is given to the heart. The patient may or may not be allowed to feed himself at first, and may be allowed to wash his face and hands, but everything else must be done for him. The diet will be carefully regulated so that, at first, bulk and fluid are reduced.

Improving the function of the myocardium at first is done by giving oxygen so that the muscle fibres do not degenerate further through lack of oxygen. In severe cases intermittent positive pressure breathing may be used to reduce the venous return to the heart. This would be progressed to active breathing exercises, then including the smaller muscles of the feet and legs. Gradual progression is made until the larger trunk muscles are included and eventually activities such as getting out of bed, walking a short distance at first, then further. A graded progressive scheme of exercises may be used following discharge to try to increase the myocardial tolerance and prevent the patient becoming a cardiac invalid.

Digitalis helps to increase the force of contraction and reduce the atrioventricular conducting rate. This improves the coronary and peripheral blood flow. The increase in renal blood flow that results, and the use of diuretics, help reduce oedema. This lowers venous pressure: consequently arterial and pulmonary pressure reduce. The decreased heart rate gives a longer diastolic phase and more rest for the myocardium.

Plasma volume and extracellular fluids already affected by digitalis are further reduced by the use of diuretics and a low sodium diet. This implies little salt in cooking and no additional salt at the table.

Diet to reduce the quantity of food and fluid is necessary because there is portal congestion and consequent engorgement of the vessels of the alimentary tract which impairs digestion. The diet should be low in bulk and calories. It is progressed from a restricted fluid diet, which may be in the form of intravenous fluids, to a light diet with adequate fruit and roughage and sufficient fluid to prevent thirst.

PHYSIOTHERAPY

Physiotherapy may be used to prevent chest infections and encourage leg movements to prevent venous stasis, provided the heart condition is satisfactory. It is also valuable to prevent or treat pressure sores and to increase the exercise tolerance of the myocardium.

Chest infections and *lung collapse* are usually prevented by giving breathing exercises in time with the patient's normal rhythm of breathing. Effective coughing should be encouraged and this is incorporated with turning the patient from side to side. If the abdominal muscles are weak so that the cough is ineffective they should be supported externally.

Postural drainage should never be used in the presence of orthopnoea, dyspnoea at rest, or cyanosis. It may be modified to help drainage of the basal segments if they are becoming congested. This must be based on a doctor's decision, not that of a physiotherapist.

Leg exercises are taught, as soon as the physician allows, to try to help prevent deep venous thrombosis formation. At first brisk movements of the feet, then adding in knee and hip movements, and later abdominal contractions, will aid venous return.

Relaxation may be taught if a patient is very tense, but when the heart is in failure the conscious method of teaching relaxation should be the method of choice.

Pressure sores may be prevented by using local infra-red rays to a reddened area, or (providing the patient is not in acute cardiac failure) an ice massage to the area. Developed pressure sores may be treated with infra-red or ultraviolet rays.

Progressive schemes of exercise may be used to increase the exercise tolerance of the heart.

Pain in the forefoot is a frequent complaint of patients who have been in bed for long periods. This is due, probably, to lack of tension in the lumbricals and interossei of the feet, which will alter the postural position of the metatarsophalangeal joints. These will become more extended, thus stretching the inferior part of the capsule and the plantar aponeurosis, and this probably causes the pain. Exercises for the lumbricals and interossei will help alleviate this.

Shortened tendo-achilles can occur if dorsiflexion with the knees straight is not done regularly, or if the bed-clothes are too tight so that the patient's feet are plantarflexed in bed (see also Chapter 16).

For references and bibliography, see end of Chapter 16.

CHAPTER 14

Some Cardiac Disorders

by E. A. BEAZLEY, M.C.S.P., DIP.T.P.

RHEUMATIC FEVER (ACUTE RHEUMATISM)

Rheumatic fever is an inflammatory condition affecting connective tissues; particularly those of the heart in the young, and the joints in adults. It has a tendency to recur.

CAUSE

The cause is frequently an upper respiratory tract infection by group A haemolytic *Streptococcus*. The cardiac symptoms may appear two to four weeks later. Some authorities think there may be an auto-antifactor present, which reacts with the antigen found in the myocardium.

CHANGES

The changes which occur in the heart are primarily in the myocardium. There is a myocarditis which spreads to involve the endocardium and may spread to involve the pericardium in an inflammatory process.

The *myocardium* develops numerous Aschoff nodes: small necrotic areas of collagen tissue surrounded by histiocytes and leucocytes, which will heal by fibrosis and contraction, and interfere with myocardial function so that it may fail. Many of these nodes form beneath and adjacent to the endocardium, which frequently becomes inflamed in acute rheumatism.

The *endocarditis* involves the walls of the heart chambers, the chordae tendinae, and papillary muscles, as well as the valves. There is a diffuse inflammatory condition similar to the changes in the myocardium in all but the valves. The valves become inflamed and

264

tiny wart-like vegetations are deposited along the margins of the cusps.

Pericardial inflammation gives rise to a sero-fibrinous exudate which may, but often does not, impede the function of the heart. It does not lead to a constrictive pericarditis.

TREATMENT

This is by drugs to combat the infection, and bed rest with oxygen to relieve all strain on the myocardium. If there is joint involvement these are rested in a pain-free neutral position.

Physiotherapy is not used in the acute phase. If there is joint involvement this is treated as an acute rheumatoid arthritic joint once the patient's myocardial condition allows.

CHRONIC RHEUMATIC HEART DISEASE

This commonly follows an acute attack of rheumatism.

CHANGES

The changes are mainly those of chronic endocarditis, in which there is an overgrowth of connective tissue followed by contraction, which gives rise to valvular deformities.

The myocardium shows Aschoff nodes, and small areas of myocardial fibrosis where Aschoff nodes have healed.

There may be pericardial adhesions which are unimportant unless the pericardium becomes attached to mediastinal structures or there is severe fibrosis which impedes cardiac function.

The endocardial structures affected by acute rheumatism—the papillary muscles, chordae tendinae and walls of the chambers—thicken and contract slowly as part of the continuing healing process.

The valvular cusps fuse along their edges as organization of the warty vegetations occurs (stenosis). Contraction and thickening of the valvular cusps and fibrous rings leads to incompetence.

The mitral valve is the valve most frequently damaged by rheumatic heart disease, while the pulmonary valve seldom seems to be affected.

While the chronic changes take place there may be a recurrent attack of the original infection with more vegetations forming on the cusps, and Aschoff nodes in the myocardium.

Some Cardiac Disorders

TREATMENT
Treatment of the valvular disorders is considered in Chapter 11.

Other treatments are directed to the presenting condition resulting from rheumatic heart disease.

COMPLICATIONS
Cardiac failure is a common occurrence due to the stenosis and/or incompetence of one or more valves (see Chapter 13).

Angina pectoris occurs when the coronary blood flow to the hypertrophied myocardium becomes inadequate because of poor cardiac output.

Atrial fibrillation is a common result of myocardial and endocardial scar tissue (see Chapter 12).

Thrombi often form in the atrial appendages of patients with mitral or tricuspid stenosis and atrial fibrillation. These may circulate as emboli in the arterial network or pulmonary veins.

Subacute bacterial endocarditis is a common development following disease of valves in chronic rheumatic heart disease.

SUBACUTE BACTERIAL ENDOCARDITIS

Subacute bacterial endocarditis is an infection of the endocardium. There is formation of large vegetations on the cusps of valves, which usually have pre-existing cardiac lesions.

CAUSE
There is probably an infective focus in the mouth or upper respiratory tract. The infection often appears following minor surgery, *e.g.* tooth extraction.

The infective bacteria, often classified as *Streptococcus viridans*, are usually of low virulence.

The changes of rheumatic heart disease or congenital valvular defects are often present, and the bacteria cause further damage to the diseased valves.

The circulating bacteria and any other matter circulating in the blood become attached to platelets. The platelets are attracted to, and deposited on, the edges of the valvular cusps, which may have been deformed previously. These vegetations, formed of a small area of calcification surrounded by a soft crumbly mass of bacteria, platelets, fibrin and white blood cells, are larger than those of rheumatic heart disease, and tend to spread to the endocardial walls, particularly the atrial wall behind the mitral valve.

Signs and symptoms of subacute bacterial endocarditis are often a low grade, fluctuating fever with an enlarged spleen and haematuria in a person who has a congenital defect, *e.g.* a persistent ductus arteriosus or valvular defect, or in one who has had rheumatic heart disease.

Blood cultures, which may have to be taken frequently to establish a diagnosis, usually confirm it, if taken during an active phase of the condition when there are circulating emboli containing bacteria.

Cardiac failure is not an early feature of this condition.

TREATMENT

Once the bacteria have been identified and their sensitivity found, tests are done to find the minimal inhibitory level of plasma to the antibiotic to be used to combat the infection—usually penicillin. Consequently antibiotics given for this condition are always maintained above the minimal inhibitory level of the plasma, and frequent blood samples are taken and tested to make sure that the level of circulating antibiotics remains at a consistently higher level.

The patient is on rest in bed, and the high dose of antibiotics may be induced by an intravenous drip, which may be continued over a long period of time.

Physiotherapy treatment may be indicated, if the condition is settling, to introduce a very graduated programme of strengthening exercises for the anti-gravity muscles prior to mobilizing the patient.

If the patient is well enough for surgical correction of the heart defect, *e.g.* persistent ductus arteriosus, then treatment will be of a pre-operative nature (see page 191 *et seq.*).

VALVULAR HEART DISEASE

The valves are continuous with the endocardium which lines the chambers of the heart.

The tricuspid and mitral valves, which lie in the atrioventricular fibrous ring, shut when the pressure in the ventricles is rising so that the blood does not regurgitate into the atria.

The pulmonary valve between the right ventricle and the pulmonary artery, and the aortic valve between the left ventricle and the aorta, remain shut until the ventricular pressures exceed the pressures on the arterial side of the valves.

CAUSES OF VALVULAR DISEASE

Valvular disease may be acquired or congenital.

Rheumatic endocarditis often precedes valvular disease and is the most frequent cause of mitral valve pathology. It may also affect the aortic and tricuspid valves.

Subacute bacterial endocarditis may add to the damage already caused by rheumatic endocarditis, or its effect may be superimposed on congenital lesions.

Syphilis may affect the aortic valve.

Congenital lesions usually affect the pulmonary valve, and also may affect the aortic and tricuspid valves.

Trauma will occasionally rupture a cusp of a valve.

PATHOLOGY OF VALVULAR DISEASE

Rheumatic endocarditis involves the endocardium and the valves—ring, cusps and chordae tendinae—to a greater or lesser extent. It causes inflammatory changes and the structures involved will fibrose and shrink. Wart-like vegetations of platelets and fibrin form along the edges of the valvular cusps. These warts gradually become part of the valve and add to its structural distortion. The repair process may take place over a period of years.

Subacute bacterial endocarditis usually attacks previously diseased or congenitally defective valves. There is an endocarditis and further inflammation of the valves, but this time the warty vegetation is formed by septic foci containing the organism which has caused the infection.

The inflammatory disease process may lead to stenosis or incompetence or a combination of the two. The other coats of the heart may be affected also.

Stenosis is the thickening and fusion of the valve's cusps leading to an overall reduction in the cross-sectional area of its open orifice. The chamber behind the stenosis will dilate and then hypertrophy in response to a greater volume of blood.

Incompetence is the ineffective closure of a valve due to distortion, contraction, and fusion of the valves and in disease of rheumatic origin the chordae tendinae will also contract and fibrose. During systole, blood regurgitates through the unclosed valve. There will be an initial dilatation, and hypertrophy of the chambers behind the incompetent valve. As the volume of blood passing through the valve increases, the same sequence of events occurs distally—first dilatation followed by hypertrophy of the muscular wall, and eventually failure.

Disease of the Mitral Valve

CAUSE

Rheumatic endocarditis is the usual cause of mitral valve disease. The affected cusps will be thicker and stiffer than normal and may be calcified. The orifice will be narrower (stenosis), and may not shut (incompetence). If the ring and the chordae tendinae are contracted this will increase the incompetence.

Mitral stenosis leads to dilatation and hypertrophy of the left atrium due to the increased volume of blood in the atrial chamber. The back pressure caused by the stenosis will eventually cause pulmonary congestion and hypertension (see page 258) and then an increased volume of blood in the right ventricle. The right ventricle responds by dilating, and then hypertrophies until eventually there is right-sided heart failure. Atrial fibrillation is often present with this condition.

Mitral incompetence, where the mitral valve fails to close during ventricular systole, allows regurgitation of blood to the left atrium. This will dilate and hypertrophy forcing more blood through to the left ventricle, which will respond by dilating, then hypertrophying and eventually going into failure.

SYMPTOMS OF MITRAL VALVE DISEASE

Mitral stenosis produces dyspnoea on exertion due to pulmonary congestion. This becomes worse, and occasional attacks of acute pulmonary oedema occur (see page 260).

Palpitations and a persistent cough are present, and there is a gradual increase in dyspnoea until it occurs at rest. Eventually orthopnoea develops.

Symptoms of congestive cardiac failure also occur (see page 259).

Mitral incompetence produces no symptoms until the left ventricle can no longer compensate. Then as failure begins there is an increased back pressure causing pulmonary hypertension, and the symptoms become the same as those for mitral stenosis.

TREATMENT

This is surgical for both mitral stenosis and mitral incompetence (see page 221 *et seq.*).

Disease of the Aortic Valve

CAUSES

Rheumatic endocarditis may cause aortic stenosis in association with other valvular lesions, or aortic incompetence. Incompetence may also be due to a syphilitic infection of the aorta, subacute bacterial endocarditis, or trauma.

A congenital bicuspid valve is sometimes associated with calcification and may give rise to an aortic stenosis in an elderly man.

SYMPTOMS OF AORTIC STENOSIS

These are absent until the hypertrophied left ventricle can compensate no longer. Then there will be progressive dyspnoea on exercise which progresses until there is dyspnoea at rest. Finally there is orthopnoea and congestive cardiac failure.

In addition, probably due to cerebral anaemia resulting from low pressure in the arch of the aorta, there are symptoms such as dizziness, faintness, and transient loss of consciousness (syncope) and, due to low pressure in the coronary arteries, myocardial ischaemia may result in angina, heart-block and sudden death.

SYMPTOMS OF AORTIC INCOMPETENCE

The left ventricle may dilate and hypertrophy over a period of years. Eventually failure of the left ventricle becomes apparent, and there is progressive dyspnoea on exercise. This progresses until it occurs at rest, and then becomes orthopnoea, and there is congestive cardiac failure (see page 259).

TREATMENT

This is surgical for both aortic stenosis and aortic incompetence (see page 232).

Disease of Pulmonary Valves

CAUSE

Pulmonary stenosis is usually a congenital deformity. It may be an isolated lesion, but is more commonly found in association with a ventricular septal defect (see page 234).

Pulmonary incompetence is usually associated with pulmonary hypertension in which the pulmonary artery dilates. This is followed by dilatation of the right ventricle leading to an enlarging of the orifice from the right ventricle to the pulmonary artery, *e.g.* as with mitral stenosis.

SYMPTOMS OF PULMONARY CONGESTION AND OEDEMA
The patient is dyspnoeic and becomes cyanosed; there is a productive cough with expectoration of copious frothy sputum which is white, pink or streaked with blood; there are coarse bubbling sounds over the lung fields with secretions in the larynx, trachea and main stem bronchi. These make an audible rattle.

TREATMENT
This is directed to the primary cause of the hypertension.
Physiotherapy (see page 261).

Tricuspid Valve Disease

CAUSE
Rheumatic endocarditis may affect the tricuspid valve at the same time as the mitral valve, and frequently the aortic valve.

SYMPTOMS
Symptoms of tricuspid stenosis are overshadowed by symptoms from other valvular disease. There is, however, little dyspnoea or orthopnoea if there is associated mitral stenosis; the output of the right ventricle is lower than normal, and so there is not much pulmonary congestion.

Incompetence occurs in dilatation of the heart in association with right ventricular failure.

TREATMENT
This is surgical for tricuspid stenosis. The treatment of incompetence will be directed towards the cause.

271

Treatment of Valvular Heart Disease

The presence of one or more defective valves throws a strain on the myocardium which must work harder to maintain an adequate output. This extra load can be reduced by surgery in some patients. Contracted and deformed valves can be repaired; adhered cusps and fibrosed valve rings can be dealt with by valvotomy; or valves can be completely replaced by a prosthesis. These operations often have spectacular results, but they are serious procedures and are accompanied by particular risks (see Chapter 11).

Conservative treatment, which will vary with the age and state of the patient, is used when surgery is not suitable or is refused.

The young patient known to have a valvular lesion may be advised in the choice of a suitable career, *i.e.* avoiding heavy manual work.

Pregnancy may have to be terminated, or special precautions taken; this will possibly involve a period of bed rest.

Cardiac arrhythmias are treated by suitable drugs.

Lung infections must be avoided, and if signs of infection appear rapid and effective treatment is essential.

If failure has occurred, rest, diet, drugs and oxygen will relieve the work of the heart. As the heart recovers the patient has to learn to live within the limits imposed by the defective heart without becoming a chronic cardiac invalid.

The complications of valvular disease require treatment and involve such methods as anticoagulant therapy for arterial embolism, antibiotics for lung infections, drugs for atrial fibrillation and congestive failure.

PHYSIOTHERAPY

This has a part to play in helping to prevent or treat the complications of cardiac surgery (see Chapter 11) and in recovery from congestive cardiac failure (see Chapters 13 and 14). The physiotherapist will be called in to treat such complications as hemiplegia, or paralysis resulting from cerebral anaemia or a cerebral embolism.

ISCHAEMIC HEART DISEASE

The coronary arteries anastomose, and there is usually a good anastomosis between the smaller vessels, which branch from the main branches of the coronary vessels, but not with the larger.

Some Cardiac Disorders

If the lumen of the coronary vessels gradually becomes smaller, the myocardium will show ischaemic changes (fibrosis).

Sudden occlusion of the blood supply to a part of the myocardium will lead to necrosis of the area supplied exclusively by the blocked vessel. If this occurs in the proximal 2 or 3 cm of a coronary artery there will be a large infarct, but if the occlusion occurs distally and the area of heart muscle affected receives nutrition from anastomotic vessels, little change occurs.

CAUSE

Ischaemic heart disease is usually the result of atherosclerotic changes in the coronary vessels which protrude into and decrease the size of their lumen, thus decreasing the blood supply to the heart.

Syphilitic aortitis may constrict the entrance to the coronary vessels thus decreasing the blood supply to the heart, and occasionally aortic valve incompetence or disease of the mitral valve resulting in severe stenosis may give rise to an inadequate supply to hypertrophied heart muscle (see page 258).

CHANGES

Coronary atherosclerosis results in patches of fibrous and fatty changes causing thickening of the tunica intima. This decreases the blood flow. Patches of calcification may be present. The changes can progress along the length of the artery. These areas of atherosclerosis appear first nearer the proximal end of the arteries and often on the left side. They can involve the distal epicardial branches but rarely attack branches which have penetrated the myocardium.

During the changes of atherosclerosis an extensive anastomotic network opens up. There are patchy areas of myocardial fibrosis, but there is some doubt as to whether these are due to occlusion of a vessel by thrombosis formation or to chronic ischaemia.

INCIDENCE

The incidence of atherosclerosis is higher in men of middle age, and is associated with arterial hypertension, a high blood cholesterol level, smoking and sedentary occupations.

Stress may play a part since men of the professional and administrative classes seem to be particularly prone. They often, however, take less exercise and eat a higher cholesterol diet than manual workers.

273

COMPLICATIONS OF CARDIAC ISCHAEMIA

Coronary occlusion results in a myocardial infarct. If the large proximal part of a vessel is involved there is a danger to life, but if the block occurs in a small vessel there may be necrotic changes which are repaired by fibrosis.

Arrhythmias occur if there is scar tissue formed which interferes with the conducting mechanism of the heart (see Chapter 12). Ventricular arrhythmias can be fatal.

Angina pectoris occurs if the blood supply is inadequate for the myocardial demand.

Angina Pectoris

This is a condition characterized by sudden retrosternal pain when an increased demand is made on the heart.

Chemical changes occur when muscles contract, and the waste products are removed by an adequate circulatory system. If they remain in the tissues, due to an inadequate blood supply, they cause pain.

In *angina of effort* the blood supply to the myocardium is adequate at rest, but inadequate on effort. The patient walks, and is halted by a pain of varying intensity. The pain starts behind the sternum; it may radiate up to the neck, spread to the jaw, and spread down one or both arms. The pain is accompanied by a feeling that death is imminent. In a minute or so the pain passes.

The same sequence of events may occur with intense emotion. Adrenaline is liberated, increasing the heart rate, and the cardiac cells increase their oxygen consumption.

TREATMENT

Treatment is aimed at relieving rather than curing the condition, as coronary artery disease is usually present.

Precipitating factors—hypertension, anaemia, and thyrotoxicosis —must be avoided, or treated. Weight should be kept down, and tobacco restricted.

The patient should be advised to avoid hurry, to rest after meals, to exclude all heavy meals, to try to relax and avoid worry and tension, but to take exercise within the limits of pain.

Vasodilator drugs will prevent or relieve an attack. Tablets of glyceryl trinitrate, chewed or dissolved beneath the tongue, should be taken prior to activity liable to provoke an attack of pain or on premonition of an attack. Alcohol is a vasodilator, and a drink at night often proves helpful.

Drugs which reduce the frequency and severity of attacks (*e.g.* propranolol) and those which reduce the level of serum cholesterol (*e.g.* clofibrate) may also be used. Phenobarbitone may be prescribed to reduce fear and anxiety.

Surgery to improve the blood supply to the myocardium (see Chapter 11) may be suitable in some cases.

Physiotherapy is of value to relieve tension and encourage a progressive exercise regime in those inclined to become cardiac invalids, and will be on the lines indicated for coronary occlusion (see page 277).

Coronary Occlusion

An occlusion of a coronary vessel gives rise to a myocardial infarct due to a thrombus, which may or may not be associated with coronary atherosclerosis.

Myocardial infarcts vary in size and severity according to the site and position of the occlusion and whether there have been any previous infarcts or occlusions of vessels.

In the area deprived of blood supply, muscle fibres undergo necrosis and the area is invaded by phagocytic cells. Gradually blood vessels and fibroblasts grow from the surrounding tissue into the area. The necrotic tissue is absorbed and collagen fibres laid down. By the end of four to six weeks, scar tissue will have replaced the destroyed muscle fibres, and fibroblasts and blood vessels will have disappeared.

If the affected area is small, a firm fibrous scar is formed, but if it is extensive the scar tissue tends to be thin and may stretch into a saccular aneurysm (see page 324) or a diffuse bulge. Thrombosis and calcification may occur in the aneurysm.

Should considerable muscle tissue be lost, the heart becomes an ineffective pump. The degree of failure depends on the severity of the damage. Severe shock ensuing in death may occur, or if the patient survives he will be unable to lead a normal life. In rare instances the heart may rupture before fibrous tissue is formed.

Less extensive necrosis may enable the failure to be controlled by oxygen, digitalis and diuretics to enable the patient to lead a normal life, or as near normal as possible.

Another problem is that of endocardial thrombosis. Lannigan (1966) states that this may be the result of the slight bulging of the necrotic area, together with the lack of muscle contraction, or that it may be due to the diffusion of the products of tissue damage.

SIGNS AND SYMPTOMS

Pain starts slower and lasts longer, but is in the same site as that of angina of effort. It is the outstanding symptom. The cause is not associated with exercise, and so rest and nitroglycerin are of no benefit.

The patient may try to obtain more air by opening a window. He looks pale and suffers from shock coldness. Sweating, giddiness, vomiting and syncope are all signs that may be present. In a day or two the blood pressure tends to fall. The pulse pressure is low, but the pulse is rapid. Due to necrosis the temperature may rise slightly. There is a leucocytosis, an alteration in the body's enzymes, and a raised sedimentation rate.

COMPLICATIONS

Disorders of rhythm may occur as there is a difference of electrical potential between healthy and necrotic myocardium. This may be a prelude to ventricular fibrillation and consequent cardiac arrest. These rhythmic disorders may occur in the presence of very small infarcts, and so the patients with a myocardial infarct are nursed attached to a cardiac monitor. This enables rhythmic disorders to be detected immediately, and if necessary treatment with ventilation, correction of metabolic acidosis and defibrillation will be used. Cardiac arrest may occur more than once owing to the electrical instability of the heart before the patient recovers.

Emboli are likely and dangerous. These may arise from endocardial thrombosis or from deep vein or arterial thrombosis. They occur in both the pulmonary and systemic circulations. The exact explanation is not always clear but thrombosis may be due to shock, low blood pressure, slowed circulation and alteration in the clotting mechanisms (Lannigan, 1966).

Cerebral emboli commonly result in hemiplegia or mental symptoms. Peripheral emboli sometimes block the branches of the abdominal aorta or the common iliac vessels and result in gangrene of areas supplied by these arteries.

A frozen shoulder on the left side is a less usual complication. It occurs three or four weeks after the occlusion if the patient avoids using the arm, and holds it close to his side because of pain. The shoulder gradually becomes stiff and painful and may take many weeks or months before it regains normal movement.

TREATMENT

Coronary occlusion is treated with analgesia, combined with rest and oxygen. Arrhythmias and hypotension are treated, and anti-coagulants given (see also Chapter 15).

Morphine is used provided the respiration is not severely depressed. Rest, essential at first, is gradually reduced over a period of about three weeks, and progressive activity is introduced into the programme. The patient is discharged home, but does not return to work for about three months. This time will be longer for manual workers.

Anticoagulants used in suitable patients, to prevent thrombo-embolism, may be continued for a period of two years following the initial episode. They are not used in mild cases and patients in whom there might be a danger of bleeding (*e.g.* gastric and duodenal ulcers).

PHYSIOTHERAPY

This is aimed at preventing the accumulation of secretions in the lung fields. Deep breathing and effective coughing will improve the venous return and so lessen the danger of thrombosis and embolism.

Active leg exercises may be used to assist venous drainage and these should be done every hour in association with the breathing if they are to be of any value; but the patient should not be made breathless, and the respiratory rate should be normal within two minutes of stopping exercises.

When patients are being monitored the increase in pulse rate can be checked without actively taking the pulse. The pulse rate should not increase more than six beats on exercise for the first ten days, but between the tenth day and discharge it may increase to between eight and fourteen beats more per minute. However it is undesirable to take the pulse regularly in the early stages of the treatment of these patients as it adds to their state of anxiety.

Patients who are sent for progressive exercises to increase the cardiac efficiency following coronary occlusions are kept on an exercise regime which is progressed so that the pulse ratio does not increase beyond 2·5 beats when tested (see Chapter 16, page 301).

SURGERY

Many patients are treated surgically with saphenous vein grafts or excision of ventricular aneurysms, and physiotherapy will be of value to prevent or treat complications (see Chapter 11).

COR PULMONALE

Cor pulmonale is right-sided heart disease with pulmonary hypertension. The hypertension is caused by disease of the lung parenchyma or the pulmonary vessels.

Changes which decrease the size of the pulmonary capillary bed (for example emphysema, diffuse fibrosis, pneumoconiosis and silicosis) cause increased resistance to the flow of blood, and so the right side of the heart has to work harder.

Pulmonary emboli from the systemic venous system or from the right side of the heart, partially blocking the pulmonary artery or one of its two main branches, may impede the blood flow sufficiently to cause pulmonary hypertension.

Hypoxia due to the decreased area for gaseous interchange, polycythaemia (the body's effort to take up more oxygen), an increased heart rate, and an increased carbon dioxide content of blood (hypercapnia) are usually present in this condition.

The patient's *symptoms* and general *clinical picture* show signs of cardiac and pulmonary disease. The progression is usually insidious but an acute respiratory infection often preludes the patient's visit to a doctor.

There will be signs of peripheral cyanosis, which becomes central if the right side of the heart is in failure. The X-ray shows enlargement of the pulmonary artery and its branches, together with enlargement of the right ventricle. The patient will give a history of increasing fatigue and shortness of breath on exertion but not dyspnoea.

TREATMENT

Treatment of any pulmonary infection alleviates the cardiac condition.

Obstructive airways disease will be treated with bronchodilators

278

and aerosol nebulizers such as isoprenaline, in an effort to keep the airways open. Bronchoscopy to clear the lung fields may have to be used, and bag-squeezing to improve the oxygen uptake.

In severe cases tracheostomy and nursing on a positive pressure respirator with regular clearance of the lung fields by suction may be needed. Diuretics are given to relieve the effects of the cardiac failure. *Physiotherapy* treatment is aimed at clearing the lung fields and maintaining a clear airway.

It is imperative to clear the lung fields as soon and as quickly as possible. Providing the patient is fit enough postural drainage with percussion techniques, effective coughing, or suction if necessary, are used. This is done following administration of a bronchodilator at the point of its maximum effect, if one is being used.

The patient may be irritable and sleepy due to the alteration in blood gases, and it may be necessary to prevent sleep which depresses respiration, and actively encourage coughing every one or two hours.

If bag-squeezing is being used then treatment should be synchronized with this event.

For treatment on a respirator (see Chapter 4).

HYPERTENSION

This is the persistent elevation of the arterial blood pressure above the accepted upper limit of 160/90 mm Hg.

Benign hypertension may be primary or essential hypertension of an unknown origin, or secondary hypertension due to a known pathological process, usually acute or chronic nephritis.

Malignant hypertension may be primary or secondary in nature. It is a rapidly progressive form which occurs mainly amongst men.

Hypertension produces a consistently high arterial pressure during the systolic and diastolic phases of the cardiac cycle, because there is an increased peripheral resistance to the flow of blood through the arterioles. The increased peripheral resistance in secondary hypertension is due to a pressor substance secreted by the damaged kidney.

Coarctation of the aorta will produce a high blood pressure reading during the systolic phase only.

Men and women of middle age are affected by hypertension. Essential hypertension appears between the fifth and seventh decade, while secondary hypertension usually occurs before the fourth decade. Hypertension occurs more frequently in countries with high living standards and may be associated with conditions of stress.

Pathological changes occur in the heart and blood vessels. The left ventricle's response to a greater resistance is hypertrophy, and, eventually, failure. Atheroma (fatty degeneration) of the coronary arteries and coronary arterial insufficiency cause further cardiac symptoms. Increased peripheral resistance places a lateral strain on the walls of all the arteries and consequently they show arterio-sclerotic changes. In the large and middle-sized arteries atheromatous changes occur. These changes increase the arterial resistance to blood flow.

Malignant hypertension, in which the blood pressure is very high, shows more extensive degeneration of the arterioles, particularly those of the kidneys and the retina of the eye.

Signs and symptoms of benign hypertension may not be present in a large number of cases (99 %). The physical signs will usually be due to too much mechanical strain on the left ventricle which will hypertrophy, and eventually become insufficient. This will cause dyspnoea on effort, progressing to dyspnoea at rest and eventually orthopnoea. Cardiac asthma is often present. Back pressure builds up through the pulmonary circulation to the right side of the heart and a cough and susceptibility to infections of the lung become part of the overall picture.

Malignant hypertension affects the alveoli of the kidneys to a greater extent than benign hypertension, and renal failure occurs. Headaches, dizziness and failing vision are frequent symptoms. This condition is fatal within a year unless treated.

Complications of hypertension are cerebral haemorrhage and cardiac infarction, both of which may be fatal.

TREATMENT

Treatment aims at reducing the diastolic pressure to a normal upper limit of 90 mm Hg in the standing position.

Drugs which lower the blood pressure are used and carefully monitored until the right level for the patient has been found. If the blood pressure drops too low at the point of maximum effect of the drug being used, causing a postural hypotension, the standing normal level may have to be left higher than 90 mm Hg.

Mild hypotensive drugs may be used in association with diuretics and in addition sodium restriction may be imposed for short periods.

In the presence of severe kidney damage haemodialysis and a kidney transplant are used as final measures.

Physiotherapy to prevent chest infections or treat the resulting hemiparesis may be used.

All forms of exercise will cause a marked fall in blood pressure if the drug being used is an adrenergic blocking drug, *e.g.* guanethidine, as there will be no vasoconstriction taking place. If the patient complains of giddiness and tends to fall, exercises should stop immediately and the patient be placed in a horizontal position and the foot of the bed raised if necessary to facilitate an arterial supply to the brain.

If the patient is to have renal surgery then it is important to institute a pre-operative routine to clear the lung fields as much as possible, and to maintain this state following surgery. Eventually general strengthening exercises will be added for all muscle groups.

For references and bibliography, see end of Chapter 16.

CHAPTER 15

Treatment of Cardiac Conditions by Physiotherapy

by E. A. BEAZLEY, M.C.S.P., DIP.T.P.

The importance of physiotherapy in the treatment of chest conditions has been accepted and established over a period of years. The treatment of congestive cardiac failure entails the treatment of pulmonary congestion as the cardiac and respiratory systems are intimately connected and the congestion refers to both the pulmonary and systemic vascular system.

In many instances of cardiac disease, such as rheumatic fever, or subacute bacterial endocarditis, the physiotherapist has no part to play in the treatment of the actual condition, but may be asked to help strengthen the general musculature and incidentally improve the cardiac performance by a progressive scheme of exercises.

Myocardial infarction carries the dangers of prolonged bed rest, and in the initial stages, starting within 24 to 48 hours of the incident, the physiotherapist may be asked to start treatment. This may be developed into a progressive exercise regime until full rehabilitation has been achieved.

Worldwide research is being done to find out the effects of exercise on the heart, and its relevance in the presence of coronary atherosclerosis.

Research workers at Michigan University claim that it is known that people who are overweight, smoke, take little physical exercise, have a high level of circulating blood cholesterol and lipids (fats), suffer from hypertension and any of the related diseases, together with contributory genetic factors, are more prone to coronary artery disease. Unfortunately one cannot alter the last-mentioned factor.

There is apparently no relationship between a circulating high

282

blood cholesterol and overweight. One may be as 'thin as a rake' and have very high levels of circulating blood cholesterol and lipids.

Research has established a relationship between the lowering of circulating blood cholesterol and lipids in rats undergoing a progressive training programme on a treadmill; and on the maintenance of a lower circulating level in rats which had been trained and then ceased training. The latter gained weight but the level remained low, and in all instances the resting heart rate had dropped.

PROGRESSIVE TRAINING
Potential athletes, footballers and cricketers all undergo progressive training programmes. The resting heart rate decreases and the cardio-respiratory performance increases. The lower heart rate gives a longer diastolic phase. This is the circulating phase of the coronary arteries, so that cardiac nutrition is improved, and the heart muscle has a longer rest.

Patient Assessment

Each individual person should be assessed before treatment is instituted, so that an adequate treatment programme can be planned. Where there is a record of the patient's condition before treatment, an assessment of the value of the treatment and the patient's progress or regress can be made available to other people.

Case notes should be read, and the relevant history noted before examining the patient.

The examination, which includes interrogation, observation, palpation and measurement, should be recorded. The record should include information on the following: the general shape of the thorax, the type of respiration, sputum, smoking habits and chest measurement.

GENERAL SHAPE OF THE THORAX
This should include the comparative length, and width. Note should be made of any *deformities* such as kyphosis, kypholordosis, scoliosis, a depressed or elevated sternum, protruding ribs, ribs curved inwards, flattening of any area, or barrel-shaped thorax.

TYPE OF RESPIRATION
The *area of chest* which is being used should be observed: basal,

283

which may be costal or abdominal; apical; the whole thorax; both sides or one. It should be noted whether *inspiration* is active, as in normal breathing, or forced; and whether *expiration* is relaxed, forced, or forced and prolonged.

The present *resting respiratory rate* should be taken as a guide as to whether too much exercise is being given at any one treatment.

SPUTUM

This should be looked at and the colour, consistency and total quantity over a 24-hour period, together with information on any recent colour change, recorded.

SMOKING HABITS

These are a useful guide to the likelihood of sputum persisting once the cardiac failure is under medical control. Smoking should be discouraged.

CHEST MEASUREMENT

The chest should be measured in most examinations of the thorax, but this should *not* be done in *acute cardiac conditions* and may be irrelevant by the time the patient is fit enough to do this. The author prefers measurements taken at the level of the second costal cartilage, the xiphisternal junction, and the anterior extremity of the tenth costal cartilage. However, if the patient cannot relax the arms, the first measurement must be replaced with one taken at the level of the fourth costal cartilage which is measured with the arms excluded.

In cardiorespiratory disease the following may be present and should be noted: a raised jugular venous pressure which will be sustained if systemic venous pressure is raised, but will fall during inspiration if the hypertension is pulmonary only; *dyspnoea, orthopnoea*, and *cyanosis* which may be peripheral or central. The tongue is a useful guide to central cyanosis as well as the lips and ears. Clubbing of the fingers and toes; oedema of the feet, ankles and lower legs and the sacral area should all be noted.

The patient's previous *exercise tolerance* should be ascertained. Could stairs be climbed? If so, how many and how many rests were required? Can he lie flat? If so, alternate side lying would probably be the position of choice to help expectorate the sputum.

Patients admitted with acute cardiac conditions will be unsuitable

284

for such a detailed examination prior to treatment, but most of this information should be collected and recorded as opportunity permits.

PRINCIPLES OF PHYSIOTHERAPY TREATMENT IN CARDIAC CONDITIONS

Breathing exercises and *effective coughing* are necessary to try to prevent sputum collecting, becoming infected, or causing an area of collapse (atelectasis). In the presence of sputum and pulmonary oedema it is essential to clear phlegm from the lung fields and to improve the interchange of gases, and prevent the formation of a hypostatic pneumonia.

Leg exercises are given to increase the venous return from the periphery as there is a vascular stasis in the presence of heart failure. Breathing exercises and abdominal contractions will also help with this.

Relaxation is important to reduce the patient's physical tension, and to try to reproduce a normal pattern of respiration with relaxation of the accessory muscles of respiration during the inspiratory phase. Conscious relaxation puts less strain on a resting myocardium than contrast methods of relaxation.

Graduated progressive exercises increase the exercise tolerance of the heart. In cases of prolonged bed rest attention must be given to the anti-gravity muscles of the hip and knee to try to maintain their strength. Once the patient's condition permits, each time he sits or stands, climbs slopes or climbs up and down stairs these muscles either lift or lower the whole body weight.

Skin care of patients on prolonged bed rest is important. Sheets should be smooth, sheepskins in place, and if any redness appears an ice massage may be given to the area, or local infra-red rays may be used to stimulate a local vasodilatation and improve the nutrition of the local tissues.

Broken skin may be treated with local infra-red rays to dry the area and promote healing. If the sore is deep, infected or unhealthy looking, ultraviolet light may be used. Abiotic rays are usually used for infected wounds and biotic rays for promoting healing.

Tightness of the tendo-achilles and pain in the forefoot are not uncommon features of longterm bed rest, and should be prevented. Full dorsiflexion with the knees straight will prevent tightening of the tendo-achilles provided the bed-clothes are loosened over the feet.

Pain in the forefoot may be due to a stretching of the plantar aponeurosis and the inferior part of the capsules of the metatarso-phalangeal joints. This is prevented by maintaining the strength of the lumbricals and interossei when and where possible.

All treatment must be ordered by a doctor, and the physiotherapist should see the nurse in charge of a ward or the patient before commencing treatment. This should be done before *every* treatment.

TREATMENT OF CONGESTIVE CARDIAC FAILURE

Many of the cardiac conditions being treated medically are being treated for congestive cardiac failure (see page 261). In this case the immediate aims of treatment are to clear the lung fields of sputum and promote a better gaseous interchange, and to help prevent the circulatory complications of venous stasis.

The longterm aims of treatment will be to maintain clear lung fields and to prevent respiratory complications of atelectasis and sputum retention, leading to infection or pneumonia.

The exercise tolerance of the heart should be increased and physical relaxation taught if necessary, so that the heart may rest maximally.

These objectives will be met by the use of breathing exercises, effective coughing, percussion techniques if necessary, conscious relaxation and active exercises.

Breathing exercises may be given in any of the following positions: half lying with the knees bent to relax the abdominal musculature; high side lying if the patient is orthopnoeic or side lying if not; forward lean sitting supporting the arms on pillows on a bed-table, or across the patient's knees providing movement of the rib-cage is not impeded.

Left side lying may produce a feeling of suffocation and dyspnoea. Should it be necessary to turn the right side uppermost, a position of comfort for the patient is usually a quarter turn to the left with a pillow supporting the back behind the right shoulder down to the right hip.

Choice of position depends on the clinical picture and the reason for giving the exercises.

Orthopnoeic patients cannot lie down, and patients with signs of central cyanosis should probably remain in half lying or sitting.

Rate of breathing. The body's physiological needs establish a rapid rate of breathing in conditions of inadequate diffusion of gases. In giving breathing exercises they should be done to the patient's established rhythm, as slowing the rate without improving the diffusion of carbon dioxide may lead to respiratory narcosis.

Oxygen is given to these patients in the acute cardiac state and expiratory breathing exercises may be given with oxygen *in situ*. It should be removed for coughing and inspiratory breathing exercises but re-administered if there is an increase in cyanosis, as the heart muscle and the brain are being deprived of an adequate oxygen supply.

Inspiratory breathing exercises should increase the oxygen content of the blood. In diffusion difficulties, if there is a very marked increase in the blood oxygen level the respiratory centre depresses the rate of respiration and the carbon dioxide content of blood rises. Oxygen is not usually given during these exercises.

Percussion techniques may not be necessary if the sputum is loose and is expectorated freely following breathing exercises. Vibrations done during the relaxed expiratory phase may be used if necessary. Forced expiratory breathing should be used with discretion as it will deepen and slow down the rate of respiration.

The author finds that vibrations done over the area of lung where phlegm is collecting, while the patient maintains his normal rhythm of breathing, are satisfactory.

Clapping is not done in the acute stage of illness, but may be necessary if the phlegm becomes thick, mucoid and infected. The technique must not hamper the patient's ability to breathe.

Active exercises, which will probably be done in the half-lying position at first, will start with brisk movements of the foot, such as foot pulling up and pushing down, and foot circling, usually a maximum of five times for each exercise. These should be done every hour.

As the cardiac condition improves quadriceps contractions, alternate knee and hip bending and stretching, alternate leg carry out to the side and in, may be the type of exercise added. The starting position may progress to lying if the patient's condition permits, and gluteal contractions, abdominal contractions and stabilizations to the trunk may gradually be incorporated with the exercise regime. When the patient is allowed up, stabilizations in sitting, and eventually standing, should be given, and a gradual increase in the distance walked may be added.

287

Recording exercises. The starting position, the exercise performed and the number of times it has been performed should all be recorded. For stabilizations the part of the body to which they are given and the length of time for which they are done should be recorded.

The exercise tolerance should gradually increase, and the patient should never be made breathless by the exercises. The respiratory rate will rise but should be at normal two minutes after exercise.

Left-sided Heart Failure

Physiotherapy is given only at a physician's request. It is usually to help clear the lung fields of excess secretions following the administration of diuretics. Once the lung fields are clear, they must be maintained in this state to help prevent chest infection. As the oedema reduces and the lung fields become clear, the interchange of gases improves.

Relaxation may be necessary if the patient is very tense, and may be asked for once the pulmonary oedema has decreased and there is less strain on the heart. Conscious relaxation should be used.

Foot and ankle exercises to act as a venous pump may be requested to try to prevent deep venous thrombus formation.

Once the cardiac failure is under control a *graduated progressive exercise regime* may be started, or if the failure has been due to a valvular disorder, the patient may be referred for surgery.

NOTE ON TREATMENT
Patients with gross left ventricular hypertrophy or left ventricular failure find that left side lying, and left high side lying, give them a feeling of suffocation and dyspnoea.

If the right hemithorax needs to be turned uppermost for treatment the patient will usually be able to turn to the left, and lie a quarter turn from supine with a pillow supporting the back from the right shoulder to the right pelvis.

Right-sided Heart Failure

When the right side of the heart fails as a pump there is systemic venous congestion with peripheral oedema. Tricuspid valvular disease may produce this, and is corrected by surgery. However,

288

failure is often due to pulmonary hypertension secondary to disease of the left side of the heart, or disease of the lung parenchyma reducing the size of the pulmonary capillary bed.

Signs and symptoms will be increasing breathlessness which limits the patient's exercise tolerance; fatigue and cyanosis which may be peripheral or central; and sometimes frequent chest infections, and peripheral oedema (see page 259 *et seq.*).

TREATMENT

This will be bed rest in a sitting position or semi-recumbent position. Diuretics will be given and if necessary open drainage of the excess fluid in the legs.

Physiotherapy may be asked for to help prevent chest infections during the period of rest, and once the major amount of fluid has dispersed leg exercises may be requested to help prevent venous stasis. If the lung fields are not clear when treatment starts, then the treatment is modified to achieve this, and once clear lung fields are obtained, then they must be maintained.

Breathing exercises are done in time to the patient's own rate of breathing. Half lying, alternate high side lying, or alternate side lying, if the patient can lie down comfortably, may be used. The postero-basal area may be treated in forearm support or forward lean crook sitting using the bed-table.

Vibrations during the expiratory phase of breathing will help loosen secretions if necessary.

Postural drainage and percussion are not usually used in this condition. However, if a bronchopneumonia develops, or is present on admission then modified postural drainage may be necessary. It is done with the physician's agreement, *never* without it. Great care must be taken to watch the colour of the patient's lips, nose and ears for signs of cyanosis, and immediately they appear the bed must be lowered. If central cyanosis is present the patient should not be posturally drained. If lying or side lying is used as a position for treatment, a careful watch must be kept on the patient's colour and rate of breathing, and the patient returned to half lying, with oxygen, if cyanosis is increasing.

Treatment while oxygen is being administered is not out of place, and may be desirable provided inspiratory breathing exercises are not being done. Deep inspiration will increase the oxygen uptake of the blood and depress the respiratory centre. The respiratory rate will fall and the carbon dioxide content of blood rise. If there is a high carbon dioxide content before, this will add to the dangers of respiratory narcosis (poisoning).

Leg exercises to increase venous return and prevent venous stasis with the dangers of thrombus formation may be requested once the main oedema has been dispersed. These should be done frequently, at least every hour, and should consist of quick, brisk movements, about five foot movements up and down, and five ankle circlings, gradually adding in quadriceps contractions as the exercise tolerance increases.

Gradually, gluteal contractions may be added and, if permitted before the patient sits out of bed, stabilizations to the trunk in a semi-recumbent position, then on the side of the bed, eventually while sitting in a chair, and finally while standing before walking.

A progressive exercise regime may be requested for these patients once the heart has been rested and is no longer in failure.

Relaxation may be requested for a very tense patient. It will be conscious relaxation so that the muscle work is minimal.

Cerebral anoxia may contribute to an altered personality. These patients may be fractious, bad-tempered and unco-operative. It must be remembered that this may be due to lack of adequate oxygen to the brain.

Complications of pressure sores, pneumonia and deep venous thrombosis may occur.

CORONARY OCCLUSION AND MYOCARDIAL INFARCTION

Occlusion is due to the sudden blocking of a coronary artery usually diseased by atherosclerosis. The area of heart muscle deprived of oxygen necroses, and is replaced by fibrous tissue. There may be an associated local pericarditis or endocarditis.

Signs and symptoms will be retrosternal pain of sudden onset, which may spread to the neck or down one or both arms. There will be shortness of breath and shock (see page 276).

TREATMENT

The patient may be admitted to an 'intensive care' or 'recovery' ward.

First 24 hours will involve bed rest with the foot of the bed tipped if the blood pressure is low. Analgesics, usually morphia, are given for pain and feeding by an intravenous drip or fluids by mouth is undertaken if necessary.

Second 24 hours. The patient may be allowed just to wash his face and hands, feed himself (though the diet may still be fluids) and read. By this time sitting in bed is the usual position.

Once the temperature has settled, and the cardiac condition is stable with little danger of ventricular fibrillation occurring, the patient will be allowed up in a chair for half an hour a day, then an hour, and eventually an hour morning and afternoon with a gradual lengthening of the time. Some physicians will not allow the patient to sit out of bed for ten days, but may allow the patient to use a commode during this period.

Walking to the toilet once a day is allowed once a patient is up for most of a day. This is progressed to walking there twice, then three times, and so on in a day. Eventually the patient will be allowed to walk on the flat for short distances as often as he wishes, providing this permission is not taken to excess so that tiredness and the resting pulse rate increase.

The patient is usually returned to a main ward three to four days following admission providing the cardiac condition is stable.

PHYSIOTHERAPY

The aims of the treatment will be to keep the lung fields free from secretions, to maintain a normal breathing pattern and good expansion of the rib-cage, to teach effective coughing if necessary, to stimulate venous return and try to help prevent a venous thrombosis, and to prevent wasting of quadriceps and glutei.

The objectives are achieved by giving breathing exercises in half lying, and alternate side lying encouraging basal expansion, and using percussion, clapping and vibrations if necessary to help loosen and shift the phlegm.

Effective coughing will be interspersed between the exercises. Exercises will be introduced beginning with foot bending and stretching briskly, together with circling, quadriceps contractions and gluteal contractions providing the patient does not become noticeably short of breath, and shows no signs of ventricular fibrillation.

Once the patient is up in a chair, alternate knee bending and stretching may be added, and stabilizations to the trunk.

291

It is essential to stress the importance of doing the exercises by an explanation of *why* they are being given. The patient should be encouraged to exercise every hour, either for five minutes at a time, or told how many times to do each exercise. Three deep breaths and a cough followed by five foot movements up and down and circling and five contractions of the quadriceps, followed by breathing exercises and more coughing, and culminating with gluteal contractions done five times is a useful scheme.

Treatment is usually given once a day, and once the patient is moved to the main ward the physiotherapist may discontinue treatment and ask the nurses to remind him to do his exercises.

Stairs may be attempted at the end of three weeks in the company of a nurse or a physiotherapist, but some physicians think this is too early, and prefer that stairs should not be climbed for six weeks.

Discharge is often at the end of three weeks, and the patient usually remains at home for three months. If his cardiac condition is satisfactory for work of a sedentary nature at this time he may be allowed back. However, if there has been more than one infarct, or the cardiac condition is not satisfactory, it may be as long as eight to nine months before work is resumed.

Occasionally a patient may limit his own activities too much and become a cardiac invalid. Usually reassurance and a progressive exercise regime may be used to overcome this (see page 300).

Angina Pectoris

This is a frightening condition, and many patients become so worried that they may be referred to as having a cardiac neurosis. Physiotherapy is usually given in the form of a progressive exercise regime with assurance to try to increase the patient's exercise tolerance (see page 300 *et seq.*).

Myocardial Ischaemia

Physiotherapy is primarily to keep the chest clear of secretions and teach effective coughing and good expansion to stimulate venous return.

Alternate side lying, half lying and forward lean sitting are positions which may be used to give breathing exercises. Vibrations used where necessary combined with expiratory breathing and coughing will keep the chest clear of secretions. Inspiratory breathing exercises will help increase chest expansion, and foot and leg exercises together with all forms of breathing exercises increase the venous return to the heart.

Eventually a graduated scheme of exercises may need to be planned for patients with this condition.

Treatment will begin in the ward and may be continued on an outpatient basis (see page 300 *et seq.*).

Cardiac Arrest

Patients who have been resuscitated have sore and painful chests. This leads to reduced expansion of the rib-cage and stagnation of phlegm.

Breathing exercises and coughing are essential to prevent complications from sputum retention. The position will be governed by the state of the patient but usually alternate side lying, lying, half lying or forward lean sitting are positions which can be used.

Inhalations may help to loosen the phlegm—usually steam or friar's balsam. If the chest is very painful, external support from a towel can be used to help reduce pain while coughing.

Leg exercises are encouraged to help prevent venous stasis.

COMPLICATIONS

Fractured ribs on one side or both may give rise to great pain and further retention of phlegm. An atelectasis (collapse) must be avoided and so treatment will be repeated as many times a day as necessary, probably three or four at first. Support must be given to the fracture site on coughing, and the patient must be taught to support himself with a towel or with his own hands and forearm.

Vibrations may be done with care, the fracture site being near the middle of the hand by preference so that no depression force is given on either side of the break.

For references and bibliography, see end of Chapter 16.

CHAPTER 16

Notes on Physiotherapy Techniques

by E. A. BEAZLEY, M.C.S.P., DIP.T.P.

This is to remind students of the techniques mentioned.

Measurement of Chest Expansion

The *patient's position* should be sitting with the trunk vertical.

TECHNIQUE

A tape-measure is placed horizontally around the chest wall at the level to be measured. The arms must be relaxed if they are inside the tape as for measuring expansion at the manubriosternal junction. The tape-measure is tightened as though measuring for fitting a garment. The short end is held immobile in one hand, and the long end is allowed to move across the short end, tightening during expiration, and sliding out during inspiration. The tension around the tape-measure should remain the same throughout measuring.

READING

The patient takes three consecutive deep breaths, and the one in which the greatest difference in the readings occurs is recorded. The expansion will be in the order of 2·5 to 10 cm.

BREATHING EXERCISES

These may be inspiratory or expiratory, unilateral or bilateral, and involve any area of the thoracic cage.

APICAL BREATHING

The physiotherapist's hands are placed on the upper anterior chest

294

wall diagonally from the sternum to the acromion and lateral one-third of the clavicle, palms medial, fingers lateral, wrists extended, elbows flexed, shoulders flexed and abducted.

UPPER LATERAL COSTAL BREATHING
The physiotherapist's hands are placed immediately under the axilla with the metacarpophalangeal joints in the mid-axillary line, and the whole hand following the slope of the ribs, wrists extended, elbows flexed and shoulders abducted.

LOWER LATERAL COSTAL BREATHING
The position of the hands is between the seventh and tenth rib, in the same way as for upper lateral costal breathing.

ANTERO-BASAL BREATHING
The hands are placed on the lower rib-cage, their palmar margin being at the level of the tenth rib, palms facing medially and down, fingers facing laterally and up, wrists extended, elbows flexed, shoulders abducted.

POSTERO-BASAL BREATHING
The physiotherapist's hands are placed on the lower posterior rib-cage. The metacarpophalangeal joint should be at or just above the level of the inferior angle of the scapula.

In half lying the palm of the hand is lateral and the fingers will be medial; the whole hand should be along the slope of the ribs.

In forward lean sitting the heel of the hand will be at a lower level and lie on either side of the spine, while the fingers face laterally and caudally.

In both positions the elbows will be flexed and the shoulders abducted. In the first position the wrists will be very slightly extended; in the second position they should be well extended.

DIAPHRAGMATIC BREATHING
This may be done in several ways.

1. Place a loosely closed fist on the anterior abdominal wall just below the xiphisternum.

2. a) Place the thumbs on the costal margin or b) thumbs under each costal margin.

3. Place the whole palmar surface of the hand on the anterior

abdominal wall, the heel of the hand at the umbilicus and the fingers spreading up to the costal margin.

All these positions are used for inspiratory breathing exercises.

Types of Breathing Exercises

The normal pattern of breathing involves an active inspiratory phase, and relaxed expiratory phase.

EXPIRATORY BREATHING EXERCISES

With the hands resting on the appropriate part of the thorax, the patient is asked to breathe out. Gentle pressure is exerted through the hands in the direction of the rib-cage movement, and is increased at the end of expiration. The hands rest firmly but lightly on the thorax during inspiration and give no resistance.

Expiratory breathing exercises are used to try to waft phlegm up the bronchial tree for expectoration. This will not occur if the bronchial tube is completely blocked. They will also be used to increase venous return to the heart.

INSPIRATORY BREATHING EXERCISES

The hands are placed on the appropriate part of the thorax. The patient is asked to sigh out. Just before the limit of expiration is reached the physiotherapist increases the pressure evenly under her hands, moving the ribs in the direction of expiration. This is synchronized with asking the patient to breathe in and push the chest towards the hands, which resist the movement, gradually decreasing the pressure until there is none at the peak of inspiration. The hands move with the ribs but exert no pressure during the major part of expiration.

Inspiratory breathing exercises are valuable to increase the lung expansion and to increase the oxygen uptake of blood. They are also used to retrain a normal pattern of breathing, to mobilize the costovertebral, costotransverse, costochondral and chondrosternal joints and to increase the venous return to the heart.

If the thorax is fixed in the inspiratory position by giving resistance with the whole hand to the abdominal wall during inspiration, the intra-abdominal pressure will be increased. This pressure resists the descent of the diaphragm, and as all muscles work harder when resisted, this method of giving diaphragmatic breathing is particularly helpful.

Notes on Physiotherapy Techniques

COUGHING

This may be involuntary or voluntary. In normal everyday exercise, sufficient movement takes place so that with the action of the cilia, phlegm does not collect and become infected or block bronchial tubes.

Stagnant phlegm in the periphery of the lung fields does not stimulate the cough reflex, and may be the seat of infection.

The presence of phlegm hampers the diffusion of gases.

The action of coughing is that of taking a deep breath in and closing the glottis. The stretched elastic tissue of the lungs and chest wall recoil and there is a strong contraction of the muscles of forced expiration, particularly those surrounding the abdominal cavity such as transversus, the oblique abdominal muscles and latissimus dorsi. The intra-abdominal pressure rises, forcing the relaxing diaphragm up. The lower ribs are drawn in, and air rushes out with an explosive force through an open glottis carrying the phlegm with it.

Ineffective coughs may be due to:

a) Weak abdominal muscles which may give rise to an inefficient cough. The cough may be strengthened by placing and holding a towel tight around the upper abdomen. Manual support from the patient's own forearms folded across the upper abdomen will help, or the physiotherapist's forearm can resist the forward bowing of the abdominal muscles as the intra-abdominal pressure increases.

b) A shut glottis obstructs a cough. Short expiratory 'huffs' may solve this problem. Following inspiration the patient is asked to keep his mouth open and make a short sharp 'huff'. If the patient wears glasses they may know how to do this as this is a method used to help moisten the surface for cleaning, but a little more force must be put into it. Sometimes three or four of these followed by a cough help expectoration.

Frothy phlegm as occurs in pulmonary oedema may pour out with expiratory breathing exercises and positionings.

Expectoration is sometimes facilitated by asking the patient to breathe in and out quickly through the mouth for three or four times and then cough. Inhalations of steam or friar's balsam may help to moisten the bronchial tubes and aid expectoration. Expectorants such as Benylin might help if a patient is very unco-operative.

Percussion techniques may be used to aid the expectoration 'of phlegm.

Vibrations are done with the whole hand or both hands in contact

297

with the chest wall. Rhythmical intermittent pressure is exerted in the direction of movement of the rib-cage during expiration. This movement may be coarse or fine. This technique is usually adequate in cardiac conditions.

Clapping is done with relaxed cupped hands, relaxed wrists, straight elbows and relaxed shoulders. The whole hand is placed in contact with the rib-cage leaving the fingers in contact, the heel of the hand is raised and then relaxed to bounce off again. This 'knocks' the phlegm loose from the bronchial walls so that it can be wafted up on the current of air and cilia. This technique is usually done over a blanket, unless one's ability is such that no pain is caused by the treatment.

Injury or disease of the ribs such as fractured ribs or carcinoma or osteomyelitis of a rib are contra-indications to percussion.

If the technique hampers breathing, as it might in acute cardiac failure, it should not be used.

BILATERAL BREATHING EXERCISES
These follow the normal pattern of breathing in the presence of patent bronchial tubes, and involve the patient trying to move each hemithorax equally.

UNILATERAL BREATHING EXERCISES
These are necessarily given in any side-lying position. However, providing the bronchial tubes are patent, if the patient is lying on his right side, the right diaphragm descends to a lower level than the left and expands the basal segments of the right lung. Conversely the same happens if the left side is lain on.

The value, if combined with positioning, is to facilitate the drainage of phlegm from the periphery of the lung fields to the area of the cough reflex.

In the presence of unilateral decrease in movement of the rib-cage it may be used to restore this movement in conjunction with other thoracic mobilizing exercises.

Foot Exercises

Lumbrical action is the flexion of the metatarsophalangeal joints of the foot with extension of the interphalangeal joints. In bed this action may be done against a footboard, or a book. When the patient is up, it may be done with the feet on the floor in a normal weight-bearing position to the lower leg.

Interossei abduct and adduct the toes and work in close association with the lumbricals.

The normal tension in these two groups of muscles prevents stretching of the inferior part of the capsule of the metatarso-phalangeal joints and the plantar aponeurosis which is thought to be a frequent cause of pain in the forefoot and is associated with long-term bed rest.

Ice Massage

Ice massage uses an ice cube or preferably a ball of flaked ice. The bed surface is protected from becoming wet. Massage is given in a circular movement from the periphery to the centre of a reddened area of skin.

The patient should always be warned before starting the ice massage that it will be cold at first and then feel warm. Patients in a state of shock, patients with a dangerously low blood pressure, and those in acute cardiac or respiratory failure, should not be given ice massage.

Infra-red Irradiation

Infra-red may be given if the skin sensation is normal. A small lamp might be placed at 60 cm and a large at 90 cm from the area to be treated. Both will be arranged so that the rays strike at a right angle for maximal absorption, and ten to fifteen minutes will usually suffice for a reddened area or a pressure sore.

Ultraviolet Light Irradiation

Ultraviolet irradiation may be used to heal, to destroy tissue or to toughen skin in incipient or actual pressure sores.

Suberythemal doses to surrounding skin will help toughen, as will a first degree erythema which causes the skin to turn pink but not to peel.

A first and second degree erythematous dose will help healing and a third, fourth, fifth or double fourth will help to destroy bacteria and tissue and promote healing.

A Kromayer lamp is the usual lamp of choice if the area is small and a sterile technique should be used.

GRADUATED EXERCISES

Suggested method of recording graduated exercises for cardiac patients

Name   Age
Ward/Address   Hospital No.
Diagnosis

STARTING POSITION	EXERCISE	DATE AND MONTH 1 2 3 4			
½ ly.	F. pull u. and push d.	5	5	5	5
½ ly.	F. circl.	5	5	5	5
½ ly.	Quads contr.		3	5	5
½ ly.	alt. K. bend and stretch			3	5

The numbers under the date column indicate the number of times the exercise has been performed.

It is better to reach a maximum of five repetitions for each exercise, and if the patient's exercise tolerance is greater either add another exercise or repeat the group that have been done starting at the easiest once again, so that there is not too great a load put on the heart. This could be done three times so that the maximum number of times has risen to 15, but never 15 times in succession for the same exercise in the early stages of treatment.

The record under the date would show 5 + 5, or however many times an exercise had been repeated, or 5 + 5 + 5 (maximum).

Example of recording

STARTING POSITION	EXERCISE	DATE AND MONTH 8 9 10 11			
½ ly.		5	5 + 5	5 + 5	5 + 5 + 5
½ ly.		5	5 + 5	5 + 5	5 + 5 + 5
½ ly.		5	5 + 5	5 + 5	5 + 5
½ ly.		5	5	5 + 5	5 + 5
½ ly.		5	5	5 + 5	5 + 5

Many cardiac patients are nervous of doing 'too much' and are liable to become cardiac neurotics. It is important that they should realize how much they can do without becoming unduly breathless or feeling discomfort.

It is not possible to have a set plan of progression as patients vary from day to day and from one another; some do too much, others too little.

Assessment of the Effect of Exercise

Observation of the patient's respiratory rate, which should probably be back at normal within two minutes of completing the exercises, colour, sweating, fatigue and look of anxiety are all good guides to the effect of exercise.

Pulse taking is a definite measurement which can be made, but it is of limited value as so many factors influence the pulse, and a pulse can vary although the speed may stay the same.

Pulse taking in myocardial infarction probably adds to the patient's anxiety at first, but if used it is probably better to keep the rise in pulse rate to 6 beats for the first few days, increasing to 8 to 14 beats by ten days and 12 to 16 beats up to the end of the third week. If the patient is allowed up all day then a maximum increase of 20 beats may be allowed. The pulse rate should be back at normal within two minutes.

In all other cases and later stages of myocardial infarction it is usually thought that an increase in 20 beats should be the maximum and that the pulse rate should drop to normal within ten minutes after completion of exercise.

It will be noticed that as the heart starts to compensate again after decompensation, the normal pulse rate tends to drop, often by as much as 20 beats.

Pulse ratio is another method of assessing the heart's capacity for work.

The pulse ratio should not be above 2·5. A standard test is used— often one of stepping on and off a 30·5 cm stool six times in a minute for three minutes.

The pulse is taken for a minute before the exercise (resting pulse) and again for two succeeding minutes after the exercise has been completed.

The sum of the pulses taken for the first minute and for the second minute is divided by the resting pulse to find the pulse ratio.

Example

Resting pulse rate = 72 per min.

Pulse rate for 1st minute following exercise = 95 per min.

,, ,, ,, 2nd ,, ,, ” = 76 per min.

Pulse ratio = $\dfrac{95 + 76}{72}$ = 2·3

Classification for Purposes of Planning a Suitable Exercise Regime

The American Heart Association uses four classifications:

CLASS 1

Patients with cardiac disease and no limitation of physical activity. Ordinary physical activity does not cause discomfort. No angina or symptoms of cardiac insufficiency.

For therapeutic purposes unrestricted activity can be allowed.

CLASS 2

Patients with cardiac disease and slight limitation of physical activity. They are comfortable at rest or if ordinary physical activity is undertaken. Discomfort occurs in the form of palpitation, laboured breathing or anginal pain.

For therapeutic purposes the patient should be advised against unusually severe or competitive effort.

CLASS 3

Patients with cardiac disease and marked limitation of physical activity. They are comfortable at rest. Discomfort in the form of palpitation, laboured breathing or anginal pain is caused by less than ordinary activity.

Therapeutically, ordinary physical activity is moderately restricted and more strenuous efforts should be discontinued.

CLASS 4

Patients with cardiac disease who are unable to carry out any physical activity without discomfort. Symptoms of cardiac insufficiency or the anginal symptoms are present even at rest. If any physical activity is undertaken discomfort is increased.

Therapeutically, physical activity is markedly restricted.

A further grade may need to be used for planning exercise regimes. This will be for a patient confined to a bed or a chair.

A table of exercises has been worked out by the American Heart Association for each of these grades based on the maximum expenditure of energy calculated in calories per minute for each table.

GRADE 4
1. Breathing exercises.
2. Sitting a) Each foot bend and stretch × 10, progress to 20.
     b) Each foot turn in and out × 10, progress to 20.
     c) Alternate knee bend × 10 each, progress to 20.
     d) Tighten quadriceps × 10 each, progress to 20.
     e) Elbow circling one at a time × 5 each, progress to 10 times each.
     f) Raise one arm above head, out to side, and back to rest position. Repeat with other arm × 5, progress to 10.

GRADE 3
1. Breathing exercises.
2. Sitting a) as for Grade 4 exercise 2 a)
     b) ,, ,, ,, ,, ,, 2 b)
     c) ,, ,, ,, ,, ,, 2 c)
     d) ,, ,, ,, ,, ,, 2 d)
3. Sitting e) Hands on shoulders bilateral elbow circling × 10, progress to 20.
     f) Both arms raise sideways above head and lower × 5, progressing to 10.
4. Lying g) Lying on one side, lift leg sideways × 4, repeat on opposite side.
5. Sitting h) Trunk bend to each side × 4.
6. Walking Progressing from ⅛ mile to ¼ mile—on the level at a slow pace.

GRADE 2
1. Breathing exercises.
2. Sitting a) Alternate knee bend × 10 each, progress to 20 gradually.
     b) Alternate leg lift and lower × 6, gradually progress to 20.
3. Lying c) Lying on one side, lift leg sideways × 5. Repeat on opposite side, progress to 20.
     d) Prone lying. Alternate leg lift × 6, gradually progress to 10.

4. Standing   e) Trunk side bending × 6 to each side, progress to 10.

                f) Stride standing with hands behind the neck. Make small complete circling movements with the upper body from the hips × 2 in each direction, progress to 5.

5. Walking   Start walking ½ mile in 15 minutes.

                * Progress to walking ½ mile in 10 minutes,
                   walking ¾ mile in 20 minutes, gradually reducing to 15 minutes,
                   walking 1 mile in 30 minutes, gradually reducing to 20 minutes.

* Patients over 63 kg (140 lb or 10 stone) should not do any of these progressions.

GRADE 1

1. Breathing exercises.
2. Sitting   a) Lift alternate leg × 6, progress to 20.

                b) Side lying, lift each leg sideways × 10, progress to 20.

3. Standing   c) Stride standing with arms stretched above the head. Trunk bend to touch toes, straighten and bend back × 6, progressing to 20.

                d) Stride standing with hands behind the neck. Make complete circling movements with the upper body from the hips × 2 in each direction. Progress to 10 circles each side.

                e) Standing 3 feet from a wall in a 'press-up' position. Trunk bending forward and pushing back × 2, progress to 10.

4. Walking   Starting with ½ mile in 10 minutes, progressing to 2 miles in 34 minutes.

                 Progress to speed walking—this involves more muscle groups—starting with ⅛ mile at speed and ⅞ mile at speed with the last ⅛ mile at a slow pace. Repeat this once.

NOTES ON PROGRESSION

    a) For cardiac patients sitting is an easier position than lying, and so this reverses the normal starting position progression.

b) Bilateral arm exercises are reputed to put a greater work load on the heart than leg exercises, and so are a progression.

It is essential that patients attending for the scheme of exercises given above should do their exercises every day, but not just after a meal or when tired. All progressions should be made under the guiding eye of the physiotherapist. Patients must be trained to stop exercising if they become breathless.

In large gymnasiums there are further progressions, and more apparatus may be used.

The patients sent to these classes usually spend the first visit watching and learning, and talking to other patients who have been attending for some time. Occasionally patients will be sent to watch exercises being performed by 'cardiac patients' before they are ready to start, so that they realize what they might eventually achieve.

REFERENCES AND BIBLIOGRAPHY

Bell, Davidson & Scarborough (1972). *Textbook of Physiology and Biochemistry.* Churchill-Livingstone. 8th ed.

Best & Taylor (1959). *The Living Body.* Chapman & Hall. 4th ed.

Campbell, Dickinson & Spater (1968). *Clinical Physiology.* Blackwell. 3rd ed.

Conybeare's Textbook of Medicine. 15th ed. 1970 (edited by Mann & Lessof). Churchill-Livingstone.

Creese, R. (1963). *Recent Advances in Physiology.* Churchill-Livingstone. 8th ed.

Cunningham's Textbook of Anatomy (1972). Oxford University Press. 11th ed.

Davidson & Macleod (1971). *The Principles and Practice of Medicine.* Churchill-Livingstone. 10th ed.

Ellis, H. (1971). *Clinical Anatomy.* Blackwell. 5th ed.

Grant's Method of Anatomy (1971). Williams & Wilkins Co. (Baltimore). 8th ed.

Gray's Anatomy, Descriptive and Applied. 35th ed. 1973 (edited by R. Warwick). Longman.

Green, J. H. (1972). *An Introduction to Human Physiology.* Oxford University Press. 3rd ed.

Green, J. H. (1969). *Basic Clinical Physiology.* Oxford University Press.

Journal of South Carolina Medical Association. 'Exercise in the Prevention, Evaluation and Treatment of Heart Disease.' Supplement I to No. 12, Vol. 65.

Lannigan, R. (1966). *Cardiac Pathology.* Butterworth. (Out of print.)

Le Gros Clark, W. E. (1971). *Tissues of the Body.* Oxford University Press.

Lockhart, Hamilton & Fyfe (1966). *Anatomy of the Human Body.* Faber & Faber. 2nd ed.

McDowell (1964). *Handbook of Physiology and Biochemistry.* John Murray. 43rd ed.

Muir's Textbook of Pathology. 9th ed. 1971 (revised by D. F. Cappell). Edward Arnold.

Owen, Stretton & Vallance-Owen (1968). *Essentials of Cardiology.* Lloyd-Luke. 2nd ed.

Passmore & Robson. *A Companion to Medical Studies.* Blackwell.

Price's Textbook of the Practice of Medicine (1973). Churchill-Livingstone. 11th ed.

Sinclair (1970). *An Introduction to Functional Anatomy.* Blackwell. 4th ed.

Tuttle & Schottelius (1969). *Textbook of Physiology.* Mosby. 16th ed.

Wright's Applied Physiology. 12th ed. 1971 (revised by Keele & Neil). Oxford University Press.

CHAPTER 17

Anatomy and Physiology of the Peripheral Vascular System

by J. PICKERING, M.C.S.P.

ANATOMY

For an understanding of the diseases of blood vessels and their treatment, knowledge of the structure, arrangement and nerve supply of the blood vessels is important.

With the exception of the capillaries the blood vessels have three coats—an outer, the *tunica adventitia*, which mainly consists of fibrous tissue, a middle, the *tunica media*, which consists of muscular and elastic fibres, and the *tunica intima*, consisting of a smooth layer of flat endothelial cells on a subendothelial elastic layer (see Fig. 17/1, page 312).

The actual size of the lumen, the thickness of the walls and their structure vary with the function of the vessels. The large arteries have to convey blood from the heart to the periphery, converting the intermittent ejection of blood from the ventricles into a continuous stream. Consequently their walls are thin in comparison to the size of the lumen and contain more elastic than muscular tissue. This elasticity allows them to expand and recoil, and loss of this elasticity in disease results in a rise in systolic blood pressure.

The medium-sized arteries and arterioles have fewer elastic fibres and more muscle tissue in the middle coats so that they are able to contract and relax, thus varying the local flow of blood.

Since the interchange of gases and substances in solution takes place across the capillary wall, these vessels consist only of a single layer of flattened endothelial cells on a fine basement membrane. To serve this function these capillaries are interposed between the

307

arteries and the veins, though at various sites in the body there is direct connection between small arteries and veins, the arteriovenous anastomosis. If the connecting vessel is patent, blood bypasses the capillary bed, and if the vessel is closed blood flows through the bed. In this way a local regulation of blood occurs.

The veins have to carry blood back to the heart, and since venous blood pressure is considerably less than that in the arteries, their walls are thinner and their lumen greater. There is little muscular or elastic tissue in the middle coat. Since pressure is low and flow is, in many veins, against gravity, veins subjected to muscular pressure are equipped with valves.

Valves are present to prevent backflow of blood. They consist of part of the inner layer doubled back on itself and completely covered with endothelium. Valves are semilunar and are usually found opposite each other. The convex edge is attached to the vessel wall and the concave margin is free, lying close to the vein wall in the direction of the blood flow. If there is any regurgitation, the valves are disturbed and their opposed edges come into contact with each other so preventing backflow. On the cardiac side the valve is pouched so that when filled with blood it looks knotted.

Table to Show Differences in Coats of Arteries and Veins

VESSEL	TUNICA INTIMA	TUNICA MEDIA	TUNICA ADVENTITIA
Large arteries	Endothelial cells. Elastic—collagen fibres with plain muscle.	Elastic membranes separated by fibrous tissue.	Fibrous tissue. Few elastic fibres (thin layer).
Medium arteries	Endothelial cells. Elastic membrane.	Plain muscle cells. Few elastic membranes.	Collagen and elastic fibres. Areolar tissue.
Small veins	Endothelial cells. Connective tissue.	Elastic fibres. White fibrous tissue. Some muscle fibres.	Areolar tissue. Longitudinal elastic fibres.
Medium veins	Endothelial cells. Elastic fibres.	Connective tissue and elastic and muscle fibres.	Areolar tissue and elastic fibres.

Veins are arranged in superficial and deep groups, superficial veins running in the superficial fascia. Deep veins mainly run in the fascial planes between the muscle groups, where they are subject to muscle contraction and relaxation. This is particularly important in the lower extremities where a long column of blood has to be returned to the heart. The deep veins of the calves lie between soleus and the posterior tibiofibular muscles, so that on each contraction of these muscles blood is pumped on, valves preventing backflow as the muscles relax. This is vitally important in the prevention of venous stasis and is often spoken of as the leg muscle pump (the *soleal pump*). The dense fascia of the lower extremities makes the muscle pumps particularly effective.

All venous blood has eventually to pass deep and there are therefore many communicating veins passing through the deep fascia from superficial to deep veins. These perforating veins are protected by valves which ensure flow into the deep veins and prevent reverse flow. When the muscles contract and blood is pumped on in the deep veins, flow from superficial to deep veins is aided. Should these valves be deficient or destroyed by involvement in deep vein thrombosis, blood will tend to flow from deep to superficial, overloading the latter veins and resulting in stasis, oedema and sometimes varicosity.

Collateral Circulation

Arteries may end by joining another artery directly, such as occurs in the case of the two vertebral arteries and the radial and ulnar arteries in the hand. Such an anastomosis allows blood to reach the territory of supply in the event of one main artery being blocked. Often it is the smaller branches of the arteries which anastomose, as is seen round joints. This forms the basis of a collateral circulation, so important in arterial injury or disease. If the main arterial stem is obstructed, blood can flow from the branches given off proximal to the block into the artery distal through branches given off distally. In the course of time, if the obstruction is not relieved, the branches tend to lengthen and their walls to thicken, so that they become capable of supplying the necessary nutrients and gases to the regions supplied by the obstructed vessels.

This collateral circulation tends to develop as the years go by and the needs of the body require it. In disease the state of these collateral vessels will determine the fate of the tissues. If they are unaffected by disease and the degenerative changes in the parent vessel develop slowly, the outlook is good, but sudden blocking may not allow time for an adequate dilatation of the collaterals before necrosis of the tissues occurs. Alternatively the collateral circulation may not be well developed or the vessels themselves may be diseased and be unable to dilate to bring in enough blood to sustain the tissues.

Some arteries, such as those which penetrate the cerebral cortex, do not anastomose other than through the capillary bed. These are known as end-arteries. Obstruction of these arteries will lead to certain cutting off of the blood supply to their territories with consequent death of the tissues.

THROMBOSIS

Blood does not clot in normal healthy blood vessels. The smooth endothelial lining does not provide the contact factor necessary for the formation of thromboplastin (Bell, Davidson & Scarborough) and the blood itself contains anticoagulants. If, however, the endothelium is damaged by trauma or disease, thromboplastin is released and blood cells can adhere to the vessel wall. If in addition flow is slowed, a build-up of cells and fibrin is likely to occur, and as this gradually increases in size it obstructs blood flow and increases the likelihood of coagulation. Should the blood flow be slow and turbulent (as it is likely to be in the presence of such thrombi) the whole or part of a thrombus may break off, form an embolism and circulate until it reaches a vessel too small to allow it to pass, when it cuts off nutrition from any tissues solely supplied by the vessel it blocks. The effect of the embolus depends on the area of tissue affected and the presence and state of any collateral vessels, including the speed at which they are able to dilate.

CONTROL OF BLOOD VESSELS

Blood vessels can change their diameter. This is brought about in many different ways.

The smooth muscle in the vessels is normally in a state of partial contraction due to stimuli continuously sent out from the *vasomotor centre*. This centre is thought to be situated in the fourth ventricle. It may not be an actual centre, but a diffuse network of neurone groups in the reticular formation.

Research has shown that the pathway of the vasoconstrictor fibres is by the lateral columns of the spinal cord. The fibres synapse in the lateral horns of the first thoracic to second lumbar segments inclusive. Preganglionic fibres are the axons of these cells. They leave the cord in the ventral nerve root and emerge in the spinal nerves, leave the nerves in the white rami to enter the sympathetic trunks. Here they may synapse at once or run up or down to synapse, for the upper limbs in the cervical ganglia and for the lower limbs in the lower lumbar and upper sacral ganglia.

Postganglionic fibres enter the spinal nerves via the grey rami, and are carried in both dorsal and ventral primary rami to be distributed with these nerves. Some fibres pass directly from the ganglia to the larger arteries (see Fig. 17/1).

Most of the fibres for the upper limb pass from the stellate ganglion (inferior cervical ganglion) into the eighth cervical and first thoracic nerves, so entering the lower trunk of the brachial plexus. The majority of the fibres then run in the median and ulnar nerves, fewer are found in the musculocutaneous, radial and circumflex nerves. For the lower limbs some fibres pass from the lower lumbar ganglia into the lumbar plexus to be distributed with the femoral and obturator nerves. Many pass from the upper sacral ganglia into the sciatic nerve to be distributed with the tibial and common peroneal branches (Martin, Lynn, Dible & Aird).

The activity of the vasomotor centre is increased or decreased by nervous and chemical stimuli. Increased activity increases vasoconstriction, while decreased activity has the reverse effect.

Factors which Influence the Vasomotor Centre

Stimulation of the baroreceptors in the arch of the aorta and carotid sinus by a rise in blood pressure has an inhibitory effect on the centre, while a drop in pressure decreasing the stimuli decreases the centre's activity and causes vasodilatation.

The centre can be inhibited or stimulated by messages reaching it from the cerebral cortex, *e.g.* emotional stress and excitement increase vasomotor tone and vascular constriction.

Sensory nerves all over the body may affect the centre in either direction, thus mildly painful stimuli excite and severe stimuli depress the centre.

Activity in the respiratory centre increases activity in the vasomotor centre.

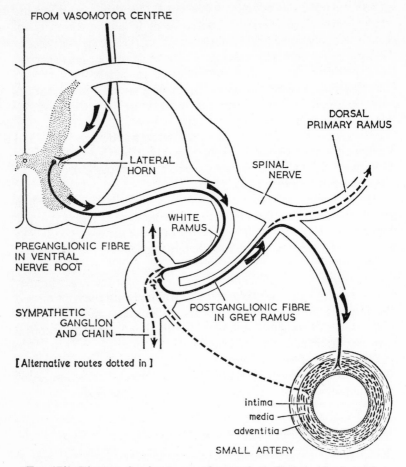

FIG. 17/1. Diagram showing course of sympathetic fibres to blood vessels, and structure of a small artery

Increase in the carbon dioxide content of the blood and decrease in oxygen increase the activity. This effect is both direct, through the blood reaching the centre, and indirect, through nerve impulses arising in the aortic and carotid bodies.

Vasodilatation can also be obtained through the temperature regulating centre in the hypothalamus. Warming one limb, for example, will bring about widespread vasodilatation since the warmed blood will reach the centre as will nerve impulses from temperature receptors in the limb. Use is sometimes made of this when trying to produce increased blood flow in a limb suffering from poor blood supply, and in which it would be unwise to apply the heat directly to the limb.

Local blood flow is also influenced by heat and cold and by metabolites. The latter are released from the active tissues, and are able to overcome the sympathetic tone and dilate arterioles and capillaries, both directly and through the axon reflex. This can be seen in the *triple response* when the skin is stimulated or a vaso-dilator such as histamine is introduced. The first stage is the appearance of a red line due to capillary dilatation, and is the result of the released H-substances. The second stage is the appearance of a bright red flare due to the dilatation of the arterioles following stimulation of the axon reflex. Finally a weal appears due to the increased exudate of fluid from the dilated capillaries. This triple response is used therapeutically to produce a very local increased blood flow.

Heat has a direct effect upon the walls of the small blood vessels causing dilatation and also acts indirectly by causing release of metabolites. Temperatures between 10 and 20° C constrict the arterioles, stasis occurs in the capillaries, oxygen is lost to the tissues and the local area becomes cyanosed. If the capillaries also constrict, the skin will become white. Green points out that in some people the blood vessels are unduly sensitive to cold, which causes long-lasting vasoconstriction. This is seen in sufferers from Raynaud's disease.

Vasodilatation usually results from decrease of the normal vaso-motor tone, but in some areas of the body nerves do convey vaso-dilator fibres. Thus the nerves to the external genitalia convey these fibres, and some nerves to muscles are thought also to carry vaso-dilators. There may be groups of cells in the floor of the fourth ventricle, stimulation of which produces dilatation. Their axons travel in the antero-lateral column and the final pathway is probably in the posterior nerve root and spinal nerves.

For further reading, see end of Chapter 19.

313

CHAPTER 18

Common Diseases of Blood Vessels

by J. PICKERING, M.C.S.P.

The number of people affected by vascular diseases is increasing yearly, and more are dying from either these disorders or their complications.

As yet there is no definite known cause, but many factors appear to have some effect on the course of the diseases. These are mainly wrong diet, obesity and hypertension. A raised serum cholesterol level and a soft water supply are believed by some schools of thought to increase the risk of disease. Cigarette smoking is believed by many people to be an important factor because some diseases, *e.g.* Buerger's disease, seem to be arrested when the patient gives up smoking.

Cigarette smokers, according to some surveys, run twice the risk of myocardial infarction as do non-smokers. The risk lessens on giving up smoking. Peripheral arterial disease occurs in only 1% of non-smokers compared with up to 30% of the normal population. Men who smoke and have a raised serum cholesterol level and hypertension, have ten times the risk of coronary disease as men in whom all three factors are absent (Framingham's study).

Men and women in the 30 to 60 age group with a raised systolic pressure show a high rate of coronary disease and morbidity. 'Strokes' and abdominal aneurysms are also more common in hypertensive patients, according to post-mortem evidence.

ATHEROSCLEROSIS

Obliterative arterial disease is the commonest cause of death in middle and later life. Men are affected more often than women, and

314

those in the 60 to 70 age group are more at risk (though the incidence in younger people is increasing). The nature of the disease is still uncertain; in fact, there is not even agreement on the meaning of the name itself. Crawford in 1960 defined atherosclerosis as the 'widely prevalent arterial lesion characterized by patchy thickening of the intima, the thickening comprising accumulations of fat and layers of collagen-like fibres, both being present in widely varying proportions'.

Suggestions have been made that the aortic intima may buckle due to the shearing action of the pulse wave, but this is not universally accepted.

The thickening of the intima leads to narrowing of the lumen and eventually to complete occlusion.

The disease is generalized, thus if it is present in one limb it is likely that the coronary and cerebral arteries and vessels of the other limbs are also involved.

As the lumen of the vessels becomes diminished, the blood flow decreases. Many people may not notice this because their normal activity is low, but the more active person will feel the effects of ischaemia during exercise. Eventually, as flow continues to decrease, a level may be reached when the area becomes ischaemic even at rest, and at this stage nutrition may be inadequate to maintain life of the tissues and gangrene may develop.

Intermittent Claudication

The symptom which usually causes a patient to seek medical advice is pain. This is initially pain on exercise though later it becomes 'rest pain'. Pain occurs in the region supplied by the affected artery after a regular amount of work of a given group of muscles, and is relieved by rest. It develops again on repetition of that amount of work. As the disease progresses so pain develops on a decreased amount of exercise. Thus a patient may be able to walk 100 yards before the onset of pain in the calf. This forces him to stand still, when the pain subsides. Gradually the distance he can walk before pain forces him to stop decreases. The pain is usually described as cramp-like or as a tight feeling in the calf which causes limping.

The most common site for block is at the femoro-popliteal junction, but changes may occur at other sites (see Fig. 18/1), when the symptoms produced are not so immediately obvious and may lead to

315

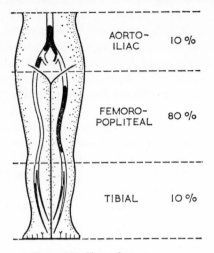

FIG. 18/1. Sites of aneurysms

confusion in diagnosis. Thus an aorto-iliac block may appear as backache and an anterior tibial artery block as foot strain.

The explanation of intermittent claudication lies in the fact that, in walking, gastrocnemius and soleus need extra blood, and if the vessels are normal the arterial bed in the muscles becomes wide open to supply the need and avoid ischaemia. The pressure in the normal vessels maintains the bed open during the pause in which the muscles relax. If the vessels are diseased and the blood supply deficient, the pressure will not be adequate to perfuse the muscles. Hyperaemia and post-exercise inflow are smaller and slower than in normal vessels.

Almost all people who present with intermittent claudication have at least one absent pulse.

From follow-ups on patients suffering from intermittent claudication, it has been found that they are more likely to die or become seriously disabled from atherosclerosis of the coronary or cerebral arteries than from increased severity of the disease in the peripheral vessels or from loss of a limb. Over 50% of the patients die from myocardial infarcts, the next highest group being 14% from cerebrovascular accidents.

Rest pain develops when the resting blood level is lower than is

316

needed for adequate perfusion. During sleep there is widespread vasodilatation of the whole body, with gradual shunting of blood away from the affected limb. The pain threshold is eventually reached, the patient wakes up in pain and hangs the leg over the side of the bed to refill the blood vessels. At this stage skin changes begin to appear and nail growth slows down. These symptoms may be relieved by sympathectomy or by reconstructive surgery where possible.

As the disease progresses, muscle wasting and gangrene may occur. Gangrene may well be confined to a small area over a pressure point. If there is a localized arterial block ulcers may develop at the site, which will only heal if they are kept completely sterile and the nutrition to the area is increased.

BUERGER'S DISEASE

There is some doubt as to whether this disease does exist as a separate entity. Certainly a disease in which the distal vessels become inflamed, thrombosed and eventually obliterated does exist. This is a disease in which cigarette smoking is thought to be one of the main causes. If the patient can be persuaded to stop smoking, the progress of the disease is slowed down and may practically stop.

Both arms and legs may be affected, although usually the disease starts in the vessels of one limb. Even with incipient gangrene, the pulses are usually present but rest pain is a feature and is often acute. The distal areas of the limbs are red and the nails deformed. As the disease becomes chronic, the skin appears thin and the toes become blue.

Treatment

Reconstructive surgery may be possible in the very early stages if there is a localized block. Later it may not be possible because all the distal vessels are affected and no suitable vessels can be found to which a graft can be joined. Sympathectomy then seems to give the best relief. Conservative treatment is usually the initial form of treatment and has three main objects.

Firstly it is necessary to stop smoking. This may produce withdrawal symptoms and tranquillizers and pain-killing injections may be necessary.

317

Secondly the risk of thrombosis is reduced by the use of anti-coagulants.

Encouraging the sterility of the area is a *third object*. This is important because if the area is not sterile and an amputation becomes necessary the wound will fail to heal. Systemic antibiotics and local hygiene are essential means of treatment.

ARTERIAL THROMBOSIS AND EMBOLISM

A thrombus is a solid body forming within a blood vessel where there is some irregularity in the vessel wall. The lumen of the vessel may be widened or narrowed or there may be an atheromatous irregularity. The thrombus consists of platelets and leucocytes with fibrin and red cells. It may occlude the whole artery so that the only blood flow in the part is through collaterals, and these vessels may themselves eventually become affected by atherosclerosis.

Should a part or the whole of the thrombus become detached before it completely blocks the vessel, it becomes an embolus and will eventually lodge at the bifurcation of, or block, a smaller vessel.

Signs and Symptoms

Sir Thomas Lewis stated that there is no difference in the symptomology of embolic and thrombotic obstruction of an artery. With few exceptions the manifestations and symptoms of both forms of obstruction are the direct or indirect results of limb ischaemia. Usually there is a feeling of numbness followed by the onset of pain on movement. The limb is pale and cold and the superficial veins are collapsed showing as thin blue lines. With a few exceptions the pulses will be absent. There is often hyperaesthesia and muscle weakness is usually present.

Table of Recognition of Sites of Emboli

SIGNS AND SYMPTOMS	BIFURCATION OF AORTA	BIFURCATION OF ILIAC ARTERY	BIFURCATION OF COMMON FEMORAL ARTERY	BIFURCATION OF POPLITEAL ARTERY
Pain	Mainly whole of lower extremities	Mainly whole of lower extremities	Foot and leg below knee	Foot, calf, ankle
Numbness	Legs, thighs	Leg, thigh	Foot, ankle	Foot, ankle, lower $\frac{1}{3}$ of leg
Cold as symptom	Entire lower extremity (Bil.)	Entire lower extremity	Leg, lower part of thigh	Leg
Paraesthesia	Legs	Leg	Foot, ankle	Foot, ankle, calf
Pulses	None below aorta	None below aorta on affected side	None below common femoral artery	None below femoral artery
Mottling Pallor	Both extremities, lower abdomen, trunk	Lower extremity to groin	Lower extremity to upper $\frac{1}{3}$ of thigh	Foot, ankle, leg
Cold as sign	Groins	To groin	Nearly to knee	Knee
Hyperaesthesia	Legs	Leg	Foot and sometimes ankle	Foot, ankle, lower $\frac{1}{3}$ of leg
Weakness	Hips, lower extremities	Lower extremity	Foot, ankle	Foot, ankle, knee
Paralysis	Thighs, legs, feet	Leg and foot	Toes, sometimes foot or ankle	Toes and foot

An embolus may show as extensive ischaemia of the distal part of the limb, and operation will be imperative or the limb will die from lack of nutrition and accumulation of metabolites.

Detection of Thrombi

It is only during the last few years that methods of early detection of thrombi have been reliable. The methods used are ultrasound, ^{125}I labelled fibrinogen and emergency phlebography.

ULTRASOUND

Thrombi in main vessels are easily diagnosed by this method but diagnosis is not so accurate if thrombosis occurs in small arteries. As early as 1842 it was stated that the frequency of sound emitted from a moving object varies with the velocity of the object. The flow detector, known as the 'Doppler', is now used in many arterial centres for recording blood flow in limbs. Blood velocity is interpreted by the difference in pitch of the transmitted sound. Readings are taken before exercise, immediately after and again after two and five minutes. In a normal person the resting systolic pressure in the brachial artery and arteries at the ankle does not alter significantly after walking on a treadmill for a given period of time. In peripheral vascular disease there is a drop in the pressure in the arteries at the ankle and the instrument can record this. It can be estimated whether adequate collateral vessels have been built up or not.

Patency of a new graft can be monitored by frequent measurements of the pressure at the ankle.

^{125}I LABELLED FIBRINOGEN

This requires very specialized equipment and operators, so is not yet in common use, but some centres are rapidly developing this procedure. Small amounts of thrombi can be detected which are too small to be diagnosed by any other method.

Patients who are considered at risk or who have slight evidence of thrombosis are subjected to the following regime. The legs and perhaps lower trunk are marked at regular intervals with an indelible marker. A measured amount of intravenous potassium iodide is given, which is followed half an hour later by radioactive fibrinogen, also given intravenously.

The limbs are scanned on the marks with the ultrasound machine on alternate days for as long as is considered necessary. Potassium iodide tablets are given daily for three weeks to prevent the thyroid uptake of fibrinogen and to prevent myxoedema.

The readings on the ultrasound machine will be high if there is a large amount of fibrinogen in any area. If a high reading does occur the scanning is repeated the next day to check and a booster dose of fibrinogen may sometimes be given.

By this method small clots can be diagnosed early and treated if it is considered necessary.

PHLEBOGRAPHY

Venous obstructions can be accurately localized and demonstrated by phlebography. 'Conray 280', an opaque medium, is infused into the deep veins (the superficial veins being occluded by a tourniquet round the leg just above the malleoli). The medium flows round the thrombus, which shows up as a filling defect at the vessel wall. If the vessel is completely blocked the contrast material will be unable to flow and will pass through the venae comitantes instead, showing up the block as a complete absence of the main vessel.

Treatment

This may be by anticoagulants or surgery.

ANTICOAGULANT THERAPY

This can be used either prophylactically for those known to be at risk, or therapeutically when the condition has already developed.

Patients at risk are those who have had previous evidence of thrombosis and who, for some reason, have to undergo a period of prolonged inactivity. Elderly people who have sustained a fracture of the femur appear to be liable to develop a thrombosis.

All patients on anticoagulants need constant blood tests to keep a check on the prothrombin level against the amount of anticoagulant needed.

Many doctors use anticoagulants at the first clinical sign of thrombosis. The drug is given intravenously initially and later orally.

There is a considerable difference of opinion as to whether the patient should move the affected part immediately or wait for a few days until the prothrombin time is adequate. The physiotherapist will work according to the wishes of the particular physician or surgeon.

321

SURGERY

Rheumatic heart disease, subacute bacterial endocarditis and peripheral arterial disease are the most usual diseases to be complicated by embolism.

Should embolism occur, the survival of the limb is determined by the rate at which blood flow through the limb returns, either by opening up of collaterals or by surgical intervention. Some patients may never develop a collateral circulation and gangrene occurs, together with evidence of deep vein thrombosis, showing that the circulation through the limb has completely failed.

Embolectomy, if the patient is suitable, should be performed within 6 to 10 hours of onset if a good result is to be achieved. Should an embolus occur immediately after aortic surgery, removal must be immediate as the leg arteries have been clamped during the operation. This means that they are to a certain extent ischaemic before the embolus occurs, and a delay in operating is therefore dangerous.

In most of the reported series, femoral emboli are the most common, followed by involvement of the iliac arteries, and by embolism at the aortic bifurcation.

The force of the pulse may break up a saddle embolism (one sitting astride a bifurcation) into two separate emboli, causing bilateral symptoms (see Fig. 18/2).

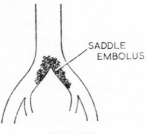

FIG. 18/2

RAYNAUD'S DISEASE

This disease is characterized by spasm of the digital arterioles. Raynaud himself did not actually describe a disease as such but rather a syndrome of intermittent claudication which occurs after subjection to cold. The cause of primary disease is not fully known but it may be hereditary. The incidence is greater in females and in cool damp climates.

The spasm of the digital arterioles causes capillary flow to cease so that the fingers or toes go white and numb. As the spasm disappears there is a reactive hyperaemia, the colour of the fingers changes from blue to red, they throb, and the patient experiences 'pins and needles'. In some patients as the disease advances, the spasm fails to relax completely and in the course of time actual necrosis of the finger-tips may develop.

Similar phenomena may occur in diseases such as arteriosclerosis, embolism, cervical rib, and in connective tissue and blood diseases and may be known as secondary phenomena.

Whether the disease is primary or secondary, the main feature is the intermittent appearance of the symptoms with progressive ischaemia leading to necrosis.

Treatment is mainly preventative. The extremities must be kept warm. Vasodilator drugs are sometimes helpful. Should the symptoms be severe and nutrition to the fingers and toes become inadequate, sympathectomy may be undertaken.

ANEURYSM

An aneurysm is defined as a localized swelling of a pulsating vessel. Aneurysms were first recognized as long ago as the second century, but it was only in the latter half of this century that replacement grafts began to be undertaken (see page 341) and since that time treatment by such surgery has become a more common practice.

FALSE ANEURYSMS   (Fig. 18/3, p. 324)
These are due to damage to the artery either in surgery or by direct injury. Bleeding occurs and continues until the pressure of blood in the haematoma equals that of the artery. The haematoma organizes and gradually a central cavity communicating with the lumen of the artery develops. This cavity becomes lined with endothelium continuous with that of the damaged vessel.

TRUE ANEURYSMS   (Fig. 18/3, p. 324)
These are mainly the result of vascular disease, most commonly atherosclerosis. The weakened arterial wall gradually dilates with

consequent thinning of all its coats. This dilatation may be saccular or fusiform in shape (see Fig. 18/3). It can occur in any artery but those most usually affected are the aorta and popliteal arteries.

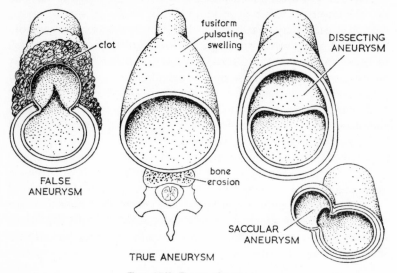

FIG. 18/3. Types of aneurysm

Symptoms

Some aneurysms give rise to negligible symptoms. The artery concerned may widen over a long distance so that the upper and lower limits are often difficult to assess prior to surgery. This type of aneurysm is more common in the older patient in whom activity is gradually lessening and consequently it may remain undetected.

When symptoms do occur they are usually the result of pressure. The aneurysm may actually press on the branches, obstructing the blood flow. This is often observed when the popliteal artery is involved, and it may result in ischaemia and gangrene in the foot. Adjacent veins may be compressed giving rise to venous stasis, oedema and thrombosis. A pulsating sac pressing on bone may cause erosion, thus a thoracic or abdominal aortic aneurysm may destroy a vertebra and paraplegia may result. Pressure on neighbouring nerves will cause pain and muscular weakness.

Many patients however do not present until the aneurysm is in danger of rupturing.

Diagnosis

There is usually a pulsating mass which can be painless or may give rise to symptoms due to pressure.

Plain X-rays may show in a lateral view erosion of bone if the aneurysm is longstanding. The shadowy outline of the aneurysm may show up, as would calcification if this has occurred in the aneurysmal sac.

Aortograms are carried out if possible to give the surgeon a more definite picture of what he will find. A water-soluble contrast medium is injected into the aorta to define the limits of the aneurysm.

Treatment

Once symptoms are present, surgery in the form of excision and grafting (see page 340) is usually needed urgently since there is danger of leaking and rupture of the aneurysm. This can actually occur in a seemingly previously healthy patient. Should an aneurysm start to leak, the longer the delay the more the shock and the less the likelihood of a favourable recovery.

Dissecting aneurysms occur if there is a tear in the tunica intima. Blood passes into the media and tracks up and down in the artery wall. This type of aneurysm is usually treated by drastically lowering the blood pressure and putting the patient on complete bed rest. Very careful monitoring of the size of the aneurysm is necessary to make sure it is no longer increasing in size. In the case of the thoracic aorta, chest X-rays are taken frequently. Later, surgery may be contemplated.

VARICOSE VEINS

Varicose veins occur in many sites but the saphenous veins are most commonly affected. They are usually thought of as a minor condition but from war-time statistics over 10% of all emergency admissions were patients with varicose veins disease and its complications.

Primary Varicose Veins

Saccular dilatations develop spontaneously and often the veins are tortuous. There seems to be no simple explanation of their development, though several factors may precipitate varicosity.

Inherited structural weakness may be present in the walls of the veins. Some authorities believe this alone would not cause varicosities but that it may be one factor among many.

Mechanical factors probably play an important part. Foote states that no four-footed animal has been found to have varicose vein disease: the erect position of the human body must therefore play some part in the development of varicosity.

Occupations which involve prolonged standing have a higher incidence of the disease, as do labouring and other heavy jobs.

Obesity leads to large deposits of fatty tissue around the larger vessels and so increases pressure on the vessels.

During *pregnancy* minor varicose veins may become worse due to the increased abdominal pressure affecting the iliac veins.

Secondary Varicose Veins

In these cases the veins become varicose distal to venous obstruction. This is seen in obstruction to free deep venous flow such as might be due to pregnancy or intrapelvic tumours. Deep vein thrombosis in the lower extremities may destroy the valves which normally prevent flow from deep to superficial veins and the latter veins then become overloaded.

Signs and Symptoms

The most usual complaints are the ugly appearance of the affected limb and the aching which occurs after prolonged standing. Oedema round the foot and ankle tends to develop as the 'soleal pump' begins to fail. This is followed by evidence of poor nutrition of the skin. It becomes dry, thin and tends to show flaking. Pigmentation, eczema and subcutaneous induration are followed by breakdown and ulceration. Haemorrhage from the dilated veins is a constant danger and great care is necessary to prevent even trivial injury which might provoke skin breakdown or haemorrhage.

Treatment

Treatment may be conservative, by injections, or by surgery.

CONSERVATIVE TREATMENT

This aims at supporting varicose veins and preventing flow from deep to superficial vessels, so keeping the dilatations empty. This is achieved by firm elastic support by the use of one-way stretch bandages or elastic stockings. The patient is advised on how to apply the bandages and how to care for them. He is told to rest with the legs elevated and to avoid prolonged standing. Foot bending and stretching will stimulate the soleal pump and aid venous return. He is also warned to avoid damage to the skin and instructed on what to do if a vein should rupture.

These measures are not curative but are suitable for elderly patients, those suffering from debilitating illness or those unsuitable or unwilling to undergo surgery.

Physiotherapy is not usually ordered but many patients being treated for other conditions suffer also from varicosities and it is essential in this case for the physiotherapist to take precautions to avoid minor damage to the area.

INJECTIONS

A sclerosing fluid is injected into the affected vein. This damages the intima of the vessel and thrombosis occurs, obliterating the lumen and preventing blood flow through the vessel. Some surgeons advise firm bandaging to help the adherence of the damaged intimal surfaces. The patient is usually encouraged to walk once the bandage has been applied. Unfortunately this relatively simple method of treatment deals only with superficial veins and it carries a definite risk of thrombosis spreading to deep veins or of some of the chemical spreading into these veins and causing deep vein thrombosis.

SURGERY

This consists of ligation and stripping of the dilated trunks. Usually the long saphenous vein is ligated at its entry into the femoral vein and combined with this the whole vein may be stripped from the ankle to the groin. Usually the leg is then firmly bandaged and the patient remains in bed for 12 hours with the leg elevated. She then gets up and walks and is discharged on the third or fourth day, wearing an elastic bandage for a few weeks. The patient is occasionally ordered pre- and post-operative routine physiotherapy.

ULCERS OF CIRCULATORY ORIGIN

The legs are the sites of many types of ulcers. The most common names given to these ulcers are gravitational and varicose ulcers. Most ulcers are the result of deficient blood supply in the limb, either arterial or venous.

Venous Ulcers

In 1906 Recklinghausen demonstrated that in standing the force of the heart beat was not sufficient to raise venous blood from the feet to the level of the heart. It follows therefore that a pumping action in the legs is necessary to push the venous blood up to the heart. The action of gastrocnemius and soleus helps in this by contracting and squeezing the vessels so pushing on the blood, reflux being prevented, on relaxation, by the presence of valves.

During the first half of this century many people worked on this theory to prove that alterations in pressure in the veins occurred on walking. Smirk and Warren, among others, found that the pressure in the saphenous vein dropped considerably during walking. The pump, therefore, is effective and there is no increase in venous pressure unless the person stands for a long time, when the effect of gravity is not opposed by the activity of the soleal pump.

The alterations in pressure in the thorax and abdomen during respiration also help to some degree by the alternate compression and release on the iliac vessels. Continuous pressure would cause stasis in the lower limb vessels.

Venous thrombosis is the commonest cause of failure of the muscular pump leading to ulceration. Bauer in 1942 gave the reason for this as being that normally more blood flows through the deeper veins than the superficial vessels. When the deep veins are blocked an unaccustomed amount of blood flows through the superficial veins. These dilate and become varicosed leading to:

OEDEMA

This arises because the capillary pressure is increased and the tiny vessels become damaged leading to loss of protein-containing fluid.

INDURATION

This excess fluid clots and organizes and the area becomes hard and contracted.

ULCERATION

The capillary damage leads to altered metabolism and impaired nutrition and eventually local necrosis tends to occur. Tissues break down, tend to become infected, and healing is slow or fails to occur.

Treatment

Most venous ulcers could have been prevented. Leg exercises and early ambulation after any operation help to prevent the initial venous thrombosis from occurring. If varicose veins are present elastic support in the early post-operative days will also be of value.

Once an ulcer has occurred the longer it remains untreated the more difficult it will be to obtain healing.

Methods based on the Bisgaard treatment are most often used. The main aim is to reduce the oedema and prevent it from reforming. In addition softening the indurated areas and stimulating blood flow will improve the metabolism, and nutrition.

DEEP MASSAGE

Deep massage to the whole limb will aid venous and lymphatic flow and reduce oedema, while localized massage will soften the indurated patches and, given to the area around the ulcer, will loosen the base and improve the circulation, so assisting healing. Following the treatment a firm elastic bandage should be applied while the leg is in elevation, and the patient should be taught how to apply this himself.

EXERCISES

These are very important, partly to strengthen the muscles and increase the effectiveness of the calf muscle pump, and partly to increase the mobility of the foot and ankle and prevent foot deformity. Deformity, often an equinus, tends to develop especially if the ulcer is painful, since the patient tends to hold the foot in the most comfortable position with consequent shortening of soft tissues. Joints are liable to become stiff as oedema soaks into the capsules and shrinkage of fibrous tissue occurs. These exercises should be done with the leg in elevation, preferably, if suitable, with the patient in lying and the foot of the bed raised, and in sitting and standing with a firm elastic support applied. The patient is encouraged to walk as normally as possible, avoiding a limp. Ultraviolet light may be used to help to clear infection (which is usually the cause of pain), and promote healing.

The patient is advised not to stand for prolonged periods, how to apply and care for the bandage or elastic stocking, to do the exercises in the way he has been taught and, if he is reliable, how to change his own dressings.

SURGERY

Perforating varicose veins, if present, are sometimes ligated and the ulcer itself surgically cleaned. If suturing of the skin is impossible, skin grafting may be undertaken by pinch or whole thickness skin grafts. These will only 'take' if the underlying ulcer is free from infection and if there is adequate nutrition to the area, consequently pre- and post-operative physiotherapy are necessary.

Arterial Ulcers

Ulceration may result from thrombosis of diseased arteries though gangrene of the most distal area, *e.g.* the toes, is more usual. Patches of gangrene due to trauma, pressure or mild infection of the skin, may occur anywhere. The patches of necrosed tissue may develop into deep sloughing ulcers, leaving deep structures, such as tendon and bone, exposed. Unlike venous ulcers these are usually painful.

TREATMENT

Warmth to the limb, avoiding the area of incipient gangrene and ulceration, and rest are necessary. Sympathectomy may help by reducing vascular tone and improving blood flow and so the warmth of the limb.

If the oxygen-carrying capacity of the blood is increased (by hyperbaric oxygen), tissues may survive when under normal conditions they would not. Hyperbaric oxygen can be given either locally or generally in a hyperbaric chamber. Oxygen is given at 2 to 3 atmospheres of pressure for a given period of time. The patient is then decompressed and rested. The treatment may be administered twice a day for several days.

330

This is still a new form of treatment and there is considerable controversy as to whether it does have a beneficial effect on arterial disease.

The ulcer, however, will not heal unless the circulation improves and an adequate amount of blood reaches the ischaemic area.

Most patients, however, eventually come to amputation because the pain is severe and there seems to be only a small chance of healing the ulcer.

For references and further reading, see end of Chapter 19.

CHAPTER 19

Treatment of Peripheral Vascular Disease

by J. PICKERING, M.C.S.P.

Treatment of peripheral vascular disease may be conservative or surgical or both.

CONSERVATIVE TREATMENT

No medical treatment will permanently increase the diameter of the lumen of affected vessels, but help can be given in the early stages.

Diet

Many people may be living a sedentary life and may be overweight. These patients may benefit from a reducing diet. The fat intake is usually limited.

Smoking

It cannot be emphasized too strongly that there is a far greater risk of myocardial infarcts and death in smokers than in non-smokers. Little over 10% of patients suffering from intermittent claudication are non-smokers, while up to 30% of the general population do not smoke.

Vasoconstriction of the terminal vessels occurs during smoking. It is clear therefore that in vascular disease smoking should be avoided, since a limb surviving on a limited blood supply would be at an even greater risk in a patient who smokes.

Drugs

Vasodilators and anticoagulants have both been tried with varying

332

success. If vasodilator drugs are given orally, their effect is general, over the whole body, with normal vessels dilating more easily than those diseased and so stealing blood from the areas where it is most needed.

If large arteries are blocked, there is little benefit to be obtained from dilating a distal vessel. The blood will not flow through in an increased amount however much the arterial bed is dilated. Injecting vasodilators directly into an affected artery is too dangerous a procedure to be carried out regularly. If vasodilator drugs could give relief, a sympathectomy would probably be preferable to avoid the regular use of drugs.

Anticoagulants may help prevent deep vein thrombosis and pulmonary emboli. It is still unproven that they prevent the formation of arterial thrombi. There is also the risk that if the patient can only live a normal life by permanently taking anticoagulants, even minor surgery such as dental extractions, or minor traumata such as cuts and bruises, could easily become serious when the clotting time is lengthened.

Hygiene

Gangrene can start very easily in an ischaemic limb through only minor trauma. Home chiropody is one of the most common causes of this. Many patients, whether diabetic or not, will try to treat their own corns and cut their nails and in doing so many damage the surrounding skin and introduce infection. Again, new or badly fitting shoes can cause blistering which could be severe if sensation in the feet is poor.

Hot water bottles should never be allowed near ischaemic limbs, but the bed should be warmed before the patient gets into it.

If any abrasion does occur it must be kept very clean and dry and all pressure on it relieved.

Activity

Exercise within the limit of producing claudication, and normal activity, as far as possible, must be encouraged. Most patients are told to walk to the limit of the pain-free distance at regular intervals. This will help to build up a collateral circulation and keep as much blood flowing through the limb as possible. Lying in bed or prolonged standing leads to venous stasis and therefore lack of oxygen to the already deprived tissues.

Physiotherapy

Some patients with arterial disease may be referred for physiotherapy, though the treatment offered has very little specific benefit.

EXERCISE

Exercise to build up muscle power in the unaffected limb where possible is of value, especially if the patient may eventually come to amputation.

Buerger's exercises are sometimes ordered, especially if the patient has to be in bed for some time. Unfortunately there is little clinical evidence of success in longterm treatment. These exercises consist of three changes in position of the limbs.

1. The patient is in lying, with the limbs well supported and elevated at an angle of 45° to the horizontal, until the feet or hands blanch completely. Some physicians like the position to be maintained for another two minutes.

2. The patient sits with the limb dependent until full filling of the veins occurs, and sits for a further three minutes.

3. The patient lies completely flat for at least five minutes.

The sequence is repeated several times in each session of treatment and the patient is taught how to continue this routine at home.

Infra-red or any form of heat is usually *contra-indicated* in peripheral arterial disease. At one time heating of a proximal area such as the trunk, if the foot was ischaemic, was considered beneficial, but in the majority of patients suffering from atheroma the disease is present also in the large proximal arteries, and it would be impossible to find an unaffected area without total body arteriograms.

When giving exercises the physiotherapist has to be especially careful in handling the ischaemic limb and in avoiding minor injury, such as might occur if the patient knocked against a piece of equipment or tripped. Not only is an ischaemic area less sensitive, but even minor injury, causing slight swelling or infection, will further reduce the blood flow and increase the metabolites and may thus precipitate gangrene.

Patients suffering from venous ulcers benefit from physiotherapy. Deep massage will help to clear the oedema which is largely responsible for the development of the ulcer. Local massage will soften indurated areas, allowing a better blood supply to the base of the ulcer. Exercises will build up the power of the calf muscle pump and mobilize the foot and ankle joints, which are liable to become stiff in faulty positions. Cleaning and healing of the ulcer can be aided by the use of ultraviolet light.

SURGICAL TREATMENT

The operations most commonly met in arterial disease are sympathectomy, endarterectomy and bypass and replacement grafting.

SYMPATHECTOMY

This operation involves removal of several sympathetic ganglia with the object of interrupting the vasoconstrictor fibres and so reducing vasomotor control. The operation is followed by a higher rate of blood flow through the limb. The limb becomes dry, warmer and the incidence of infection is lessened.

Side-effects are not common but do sometimes occur, and the patient should be made aware of these so that he can watch out for and report, if they do arise.

Postural hypotension may occur if an extensive cervical and lumbar sympathectomy has been performed.

There may be increased sweating in the areas unaffected by the sympathectomy, such as the lower chest and face.

Cervical sympathectomy may lead to drooping of the eyelids.

Lumbar sympathectomy can cause disturbance of sexual function. This is more common following a bilateral sympathectomy, but can be avoided if the first lumbar ganglion is preserved.

An embolus may be the result of an atheromatous plaque being dislodged and moving on down the iliac artery. This, however, will be noticed at the end of the operation since the femoral pulse will be absent. Immediate embolectomy can then be performed before the patient is returned to the ward.

PRE-OPERATIVE PHYSIOTHERAPY

As soon as the date of operation is known, breathing exercises are taught together with effective coughing. In a lumbar sympathectomy, as in all lower abdominal surgery, there is the risk of thrombosis. If the operation is performed as a preventive measure, leg exercises should be encouraged to reduce the possibility of deep vein thrombosis.

POST-OPERATIVE PHYSIOTHERAPY

Breathing exercises and coughing are given with good support to the wound. Toe and ankle exercises and quadriceps and gluteal contractions are most important, but some authorities prefer to omit straight leg-raising as it would cause tension on the wound. After a few days, abdominal work may be added.

If the operation has been a cervical sympathectomy, arm exercises are given if necessary. Usually, however, the patient is active and does not need much treatment.

Mobilization usually starts on the day after operation, the patient getting out of bed and progressing in walking. Attention to posture will also be started.

If a lumbar sympathectomy has been carried out on a patient who has previously had amputation of one leg, mobilization will be more difficult. It is very important that the patient should wear the artificial limb when walking. This is sometimes uncomfortable because the belt may rub over the incision site, and the patient may prefer to use crutches rather than wear the limb. This must be avoided, because it puts an unnecessary amount of strain on the remaining, already diseased, limb.

When training walking with the artificial limb, the patient will have already been taught to protect his own leg by resting with the weight on the pylon and this must be continued if the remaining limb is to survive.

ENDARTERECTOMY

This operation was introduced about thirty years ago and is now frequently undertaken.

Open Thromboendarterectomy

The artery is opened over the obstruction (see Fig. 19/1 (left)) and the thrombus together with plaques of atheroma, the tunica intima and the internal elastic lamina are removed. This operation is most suitable for short blocks and at arterial bifurcations.

Closed Endarterectomy

In this method a small incision is made proximal to the block (see Fig. 19/1 (right)) and an instrument such as the ring stripper is passed along the artery to beyond the block. This is then pulled back. If it is thought that suturing the arteriotomy may cause constriction in the lumen, then a patch graft will be used. This is taken from one of the patient's own veins, or occasionally Dacron cloth is used. The patch is sutured round to increase the size of the lumen.

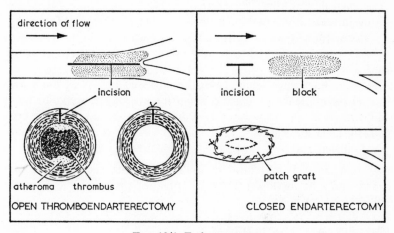

FIG. 19/1. Endarterectomy

PRE-OPERATIVE PHYSIOTHERAPY
Breathing exercises and effective coughing are taught and leg exercises demonstrated.

POST-OPERATIVE PHYSIOTHERAPY
Breathing exercises and coughing are practised and early mobilization and leg exercises given to keep the blood flowing swiftly through the artery and prevent the formation of new deposits. The exact exercises chosen will vary with the surgeon's wishes but it is usually held that the earlier the patient is ambulant, the better the result, since there is less risk of thrombosis.

Aorto-iliac Endarterectomy

The results of operation at this site are extremely good.

Post-operative physiotherapy is important because there has often been an extensive exploration and the patient is loath to move and may become 'chesty'. The chest is the first consideration and early mobilization may be delayed because of this. There is no contra-indication to coughing, and all joints can be flexed to facilitate this. Leg exercises should be encouraged, but no straight leg-raising should be done until the sutures are removed.

Iliac and Femoral Endarterectomy

Post-operative physiotherapy follows very closely that used following a meniscectomy apart from the early mobilization.

Weight-bearing in the form of 'lilting' exercises (alternate heel-raising in standing) is often begun on the first day at the surgeon's discretion. No patient should be allowed to walk until he has good quadriceps control and can straighten the knee when walking.

Carotid Endarterectomy

If the operation is likely to be extensive and it is thought that grafting may be needed, it may be done under hypothermia. Most patients are up and walking the day after the operation providing there are no side-effects.

PRE-OPERATIVE PHYSIOTHERAPY

Prior to operation, the patient may have suffered several minor vascular episodes such as visual disturbances or transient hemi-paresis. A general test of voluntary muscle strength should therefore be made. This need not involve more than a comparison of large muscle groups on each side, *e.g.*

	RIGHT	LEFT
Fingers bend		
Fingers stretch		
Wrist flex		
Wrist extend		
Elbow flex		
Elbow extend		

The usual pre-operative routine will be carried out.

POST-OPERATIVE PHYSIOTHERAPY
This should include a repetition of these tests and if any differences are noted these should be reported to the surgeon.

Endarterectomy Using a Patch

The routine physiotherapy is the same as the previous type of surgery, but the physiotherapist will note that because there is a patch *in situ* the area of suturing is increased.

EMBOLECTOMY

This operation is performed as soon as possible after onset, as the chance of the survival of the limb decreases with time.

As the methods of diagnosing the exact area of the embolus improve, so the operation becomes quicker and less extensive.

Some emboli are removed under local anaesthesia.

If a large embolus passes down the aorta it may lodge at the bifurcation and so block both limbs (saddle embolus—see Fig. 18/2, page 322). The embolus may break up and block both legs at a lower level, so requiring two separate incisions.

The incision is made at a suitable point and the fresh clot is removed. Sometimes a catheter such as the Fogarty balloon catheter, is used to make sure that the distal part of the artery is clear, or the artery may be flushed out.

PRE-OPERATIVE PHYSIOTHERAPY
Since the operation is usually an emergency procedure, the patient is rarely seen by the physiotherapist pre-operatively. If, however, physiotherapy is ordered then *no* leg exercises are given, because these might cause the embolus to break up and cause further damage.

POST-OPERATIVE PHYSIOTHERAPY
Provided the pulses are present and the surgeon has given permission, breathing exercises and coughing and movements of all unaffected limbs are started at once. If the patient cannot move the affected limb himself, passive movements are given but active movements should be done wherever possible.

BYPASS GRAFTS

These grafts are often done with little direct exposure of the diseased artery. The graft is tunnelled under the overlying tissues from the exposed ends of the blocked area.

Two types of material are used.

Dacron and Plastic Tubing

These materials are ideal in large fast-flowing arteries such as the aorta. As the diameter of the vessel lessens, so the success of the man-made fibre decreases.

Vein Grafts

If the patient has a suitable saphenous vein this can be used. The vein is reversed so that the valves are in the direction of flow and offer no impediment. Veins are ideal for limb arteries but are not suitable for aortic grafting. Both types of grafts are anastomosed end to side (see Fig. 19/2).

PRE-OPERATIVE PHYSIOTHERAPY
Breathing, coughing and leg exercises are taught. If gangrene is present in one limb, no exercises are given for that limb.

POST-OPERATIVE PHYSIOTHERAPY
This follows the same lines as in any arterial surgery, but pulses should be checked before and after treatment for the first few days. Most surgeons encourage early mobilization in the form of walking, but do not allow prolonged standing or sitting with the legs dependent.

In aorto-iliac bypass grafts the patient is often elderly and may have a heavily calcified aorta, with little healthy tissue, or his general condition may make long surgery a bad risk. The incisions are therefore kept small and blood flow through the original artery is maintained, so that if the graft 'shuts down' there is still some blood supply to the lower limbs. In these patients the knee and hip can be bent for coughing, but the position should not be maintained for too long as this could kink the graft or compress it in the iliac fossa.

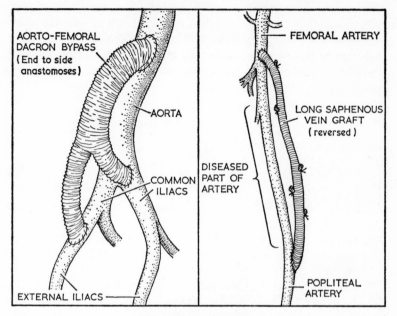

FIG. 19/2. Bypass grafts

Femoro-popliteal Bypass Graft

The graft is a long one, usually extending from the groin down to and beyond the knee. Although the usual procedure is to tunnel the graft through the leg, sometimes direct positioning is used, and in this case there will be a long curved incision down the thigh, which is often very painful. During the operation the graft is anastomosed at the lower end with the knee slightly bent. Care must therefore be taken over the first few days not to stretch the graft. Quadriceps exercises should be taught, but only within the patient's own range of movement.

When the stitches are out the exercises can be progressed quite rapidly.

REPLACEMENT GRAFTS

The affected artery is replaced either by a tube of man-made material or by a vein. Aneurysms are usually treated by this method as well as atheromatous arteries.

The artery is exposed to show the upper and lower limits of relatively normal artery. The affected part is removed and the graft sewn in between, making sure that all layers of the artery are attached to the graft. If this is not done, the blood may leak back causing dissection of the layers.

PRE-OPERATIVE PHYSIOTHERAPY

Breathing exercises and leg exercises are taught.

POST-OPERATIVE PHYSIOTHERAPY

Breathing exercises are given for as long as needed. If the graft passes over a joint, flexion is not done until the surgeon gives his permission, because the graft might become kinked or compressed by the tissues passing superficial to it.

In the case of an aorto-iliac graft, the knees may be bent for coughing because this puts less strain on the abdominal wound and, since it is only a momentary procedure, the graft is safe.

If a bypass graft thromboses or the suturing becomes unsafe, blood will still flow through the original artery, but if this occurs in a replacement graft, there is complete lack of blood supply to the distal part.

Early mobilization is the rule, but the condition of the limb distal to the affected area may prevent this. If gangrene has occurred in one leg or amputation has been performed, walking will be difficult. Consequently leg exercises will play a much more important part in the early days until the artificial limb can be comfortably worn.

SURGERY OF ANEURYSMS INVOLVING THE ABDOMINAL AORTA

Replacement grafts are the most usual form of treatment. The aneurysm is dissected out, clamps are applied proximal and distal to it, and the contents of the sac are removed. The graft is sewn into place, and the sac is usually sewn round the graft.

Wiring is used if the aneurysm is considered inoperable, because too many artery trunks are involved or the tissue at either end is too friable or the patient is a bad risk for surgery owing to another condition. About 100 metres of narrow-gauge stainless steel wire is inserted into the sac, which then becomes slowly obliterated.

PRE-OPERATIVE PHYSIOTHERAPY

If the patient is admitted from the waiting list, physiotherapy is started immediately. Patients admitted with leaking or dissecting aneurysms and as emergencies, should not be treated unless specific instructions to do so are given since the danger of the aneurysm bursting is very great.

If physiotherapy is ordered, breathing and leg exercises are demonstrated. The treatment should not be too energetic because the aneurysm can suddenly increase in size, making surgery a far greater risk.

POST-OPERATIVE PHYSIOTHERAPY

On the day after the operation, the patient can usually be rolled into alternate side lying for breathing exercises at the same time as the pressure areas are being treated. Sometimes, however, it may have been difficult to find arterial tissue firm enough to hold the sutures, and in this case the surgeon may not like the patient to be moved too much.

Leg exercises are essential, as although heparin is often injected into the femoral arteries, the blood supply to the legs may have been stopped for a long time during surgery and the risk of deep vein thrombosis therefore increased.

From the second day onwards breathing and leg exercises are continued until the patient is up and walking. This may mean sitting out in a chair and walking a few steps from the third day onwards, but it is often much later. The larger the amount of surgery, the later the ambulation.

LESS COMMON PROCEDURES

AXILLARY FEMORAL SUBCUTANEOUS GRAFTS

This is a new operation which has so far been performed on only a few patients in recent years. The patient may originally have had a graft for an aneurysm which has failed in some way, so that the nutrition of the lower limbs is inadequate. If there is widespread arterial disease, a graft may be used to aid nutrition to the proximal part of the leg when the distal part is to be amputated.

The grafts are passed from the axillary artery beneath the skin, but outside the ribs, to be anastomosed with the femoral artery (see Fig. 19/3). As neither the chest nor the abdominal cavity are opened, the patient's chest is usually unaffected, so the operation is suitable for a patient who otherwise might be a bad risk for reconstructive surgery because of his chest condition.

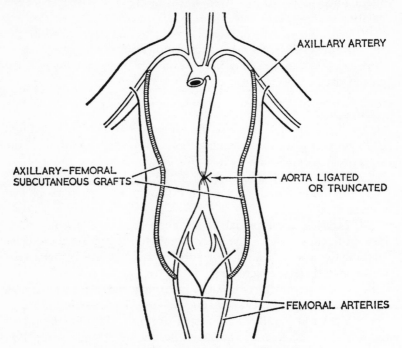

FIG. 19/3. Axillary-femoral subcutaneous grafts

PHYSIOTHERAPY

Since the operation is still very new and is often an emergency procedure, physiotherapy is not usually started pre-operatively, but if the patient is in the ward for a time prior to surgery he can be shown breathing exercises.

The first day post-operatively breathing exercises must be done with care because it is extremely easy to compress the graft. The physiotherapist can usually see the grafts as there is often marked bruising where the tunnelling occurred and there may even be pulsation. If the patient is rolled into side lying then he should only roll far enough to keep the graft free from the bed.

344

Leg exercises are done routinely.

Treatment continues from the second day onwards as needed. When the patient is allowed up care should be taken to see that the pyjama cord is not pulled tightly over the graft. The physiotherapist should explain this to the patient and suggest help with his everyday clothing, *e.g.* braces instead of a tight trouser belt.

RE-ENTRY OPERATION FOR DISSECTING ANEURYSMS

Sometimes surgery is carried out for acutely dissecting aneurysms to prevent further dissection. A small incision is made in the artery wall through the tunica intima to allow re-entry of blood (see Fig. 19/4). As the blood flows back into the stream dissection stops and the layers adhere to each other again.

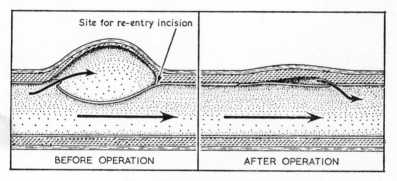

FIG. 19/4. Re-entry operation

COMPLICATIONS OF ARTERIAL SURGERY

Respiratory Failure

Deep anaesthesia for a lengthy period is required during extensive reconstructive surgery. Chest complications, therefore, may develop.

Aneurysms are usually found in the older patient who perhaps has less respiratory reserve and who may have smoked all his life.

Shock due to leaking aneurysms can also be a complication.

If these factors are taken into consideration it is not surprising that after prolonged surgery it may be a long time before the patient breathes spontaneously.

Treatment of a patient on a ventilator following arterial surgery will be the same as for any other patient on a ventilator (see Chapter 4). Tipping may be carried out if absolutely necessary but not for any length of time, because the circulation to the lower limbs may still only be adequate when the patient is in the supine position.

Paralytic Ileus

Due to handling of the colon during the exploratory laparotomy, there is often spasm of the muscular wall of the intestine. If the reconstruction involves either the superior or the inferior mesenteric arteries, there is then risk of necrosis of that part of the intestine deprived of its blood supply. This may, of course, already exist prior to reconstruction due to infarction in the area of supply of these arteries.

Embolism

When an artery is clamped for reconstruction there is stasis of blood in the distal vessels. Should a thrombosis start to form in these vessels, when the artery is unclamped the thrombus may be pushed on to block a smaller artery.

There is also pressure on veins during surgery and this may lead to stasis and pulmonary emboli may occur.

False Aneurysm

This can occur round the suture line in any reconstruction.

Failed Graft

The graft may fail for several reasons.

a) There may be deposits of atheroma laid down in the graft after surgery.

b) The vessel may collapse due to pressure on it from the surrounding structures or from leakage of blood flowing through at the suture line.

c) An infection may develop round the graft and as a result the suture line may break down.

Deep Vein Thrombosis

The less able the patient is to keep moving, the higher the risk of thrombosis. There are many reasons why the patient does not move after an operation. Respiratory failure requiring artificial ventilation means that the patient is often deeply sedated and so is unable to move his own limbs. Confusion is quite common in elderly patients or those who have had massive surgery involving the carotid or innominate arteries. A confused patient moves but may damage himself and so may require sedation.

For these and other reasons it may be necessary to move the patient's limbs regularly until he can do this for himself.

Acute Renal Failure

The shock of a leaking aneurysm and the subsequent surgery may be sufficient to cause renal failure. This may be complete or in the form of reduced output. If the blood urea level rises, then the patient becomes very confused and difficult. Usually either peritoneal dialysis or haemodialysis is started to bring the level down, and is continued until the kidneys start to function again. If surgery has been on the renal artery itself or on the aorta, then the incidence of renal failure is greater.

NOTE ON PRE-OPERATIVE PHYSIOTHERAPY

Breathing exercises are carried out as for any operation, but if the patient is very 'chesty', and it is felt that tipping would help, permission must be obtained from the surgeon. This is because the change in position might further endanger a weak abdominal aorta and lessen nutrition of the lower limbs.

Leg exercises should be taught and the reason for doing them explained, but care must be taken to see that the patient does not practise these if it could be dangerous. If gangrene is present, leg exercises of the affected limb are contra-indicated before surgery because they could increase the formation and absorption of metabolites. For this reason it is usually considered safer to show the exercises rather than encourage vigorous practising.

REFERENCES

Bauer, D. (1942). 'Clinical Study of Thrombosis'. *Acta chir. Scand.*
Bell, Davidson and Scarborough (1972). *Textbook of Physiology and Biochemistry* Churchill-Livingstone. 8th ed.
Crawford, T. (1960). 'Some Aspects of the Pathology of Atherosclerosis'. *Proc. Roy. Soc. Med.*
Framingham (1962). Enquiry. *Proc. Roy. Soc. Med.*
Lewis, T. (1949). *Vascular Disorders of the Limbs.* Macmillan. (Out of print.)
Recklinghausen (1906). *Arch. exp. Path.*
Smirk and Warren. 'Observations on the Causes of Oedema in Congestive Heart Failure'. *Clinical Science.*

FURTHER READING

Anning, S. T. (1968). 'Pathogenesis and Treatment of Venous Leg Ulcers. *Physiotherapy*, Vol. 54.
Bannister, C. R. (1968). 'Physiotherapy in the Treatment of Venous Leg Ulcers'. *Physiotherapy*, Vol. 54.
Eastcott, H. H. G. (1969). *Arterial Surgery.* Pitman Medical Press.
Foote, R. R. (1960). *Varicose Veins—a practical manual.* John Wright & Son Ltd. 3rd ed. (Out of print.)
Gillespie, J. A. (ed.). (1970). *Modern Trends in Vascular Surgery (1).* Butterworth.
Gray's Anatomy. 35th ed. (1973). (Edited by R. Warwick). Longman.
Green, J. H. (1972). *An Introduction to Human Physiology.* Oxford University Press. 3rd ed.
Hersley, F. and Calman, C. (1967). *Atlas of Vascular Surgery.* The C. V. Mosby Company, St. Louis. 2nd ed.
Kinmonth, J. B., Rob, C. G. and Simeone, S. A. (1962) (Out of print.) *Vascular Surgery.* Edward Arnold.
Martin, P., Lynn, B. R., Dible, J. H. and Aird, I. (1956). *Peripheral Vascular Disorders.* Churchill-Livingstone.
McNaught, A. B. and Callander, R. (1970). *Illustrated Physiology.* Churchill-Livingstone. 2nd ed.
Proceedings of the 2nd International Congress on Hyperbaric Oxygenation. (1964). Churchill-Livingstone.
Richards, Robert L. (1970). *Peripheral Arterial Disease—a physician's approach.* Churchill-Livingstone.

Index

349

Index

Index

Index

Index

Index